Teen Health Series

Suicide Information For Teens, Third Edition

Suicide Information For Teens,
Third Edition

Health Tips About Suicide Causes
And Prevention

Including Facts About Depression, Risk Factors,
Getting Help, Survivor Support, And More

OMNIGRAPHICS
615 Griswold, Ste. 901
Detroit, MI 48226

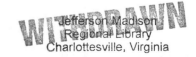

30864   5595

C

Bibliographic Note
Because this page cannot legibly accommodate all the copyright notices, the Bibliographic Note portion of the Preface constitutes an extension of the copyright notice.

* * *

Omnigraphics
a part of Relevant Information
Keith Jones, *Managing Editor*

* * *

Library of Congress Cataloging-in-Publication Data

Title: Suicide information for teens: health tips about suicide causes and prevention including facts about depression, risk factors, getting help, survivor support, and more.

Description: Third edition. | Detroit, MI: Omnigraphics, [2017] | Series: Teen health series | Audience: Grade 9 to 12. | Includes bibliographical references and index.

Identifiers: LCCN 2016059219 (print) | LCCN 2017006763 (ebook) | ISBN 9780780814905 (acid-free paper) | ISBN 9780780814899 (eISBN) | ISBN 9780780814899 (eBook)

Subjects: LCSH: Teenagers--Suicidal behavior--Juvenile literature. | Suicidal behavior--Juvenile literature. | Suicide--Prevention--Juvenile literature.

Classification: LCC HV6546 .S8345 2017 (print) | LCC HV6546 (ebook) | DDC 362.280835--dc23

LC record available at https://lccn.loc.gov/2016059219

Table Of Contents

Preface

Part One: Suicide Facts And Statistics

Part Two: Mental Health Disorders And Life-Threatening Behaviors Linked To Suicide Risk

Part Three: Recognizing And Treating Suicidal Ideation

Part Four: When Someone You Know Dies From Suicide

Part Five: Preventing Suicide

Part Six: If You Need More Information

Preface

About This Book

Teens often face a host of stressors and confusing feelings as they grow through the adolescent years. The emotions associated with puberty, self-doubt, confusion about the future, family problems, and school pressures can sometimes seem overwhelming. Recent statistics show that suicide is the third leading cause of death among persons aged 10–14 and the second among persons aged 15–34 years. But suicidal behavior is not a normal response to stress. Mental health professionals claim that most teen suicide victims have a mental health disorder, a history of substance abuse, or both. When suicide risks are acknowledged and warning signs are heeded, many teens in distress can learn that the feelings that led them to consider suicide are treatable and that there is hope for the future.

Suicide Information for Teens, Third Edition, provides updated information about suicide risks, causes, and prevention. It discusses mental health disorders and life-threatening behaviors linked to suicide risk, including depression, bipolar disorder, anxiety disorders, eating disorders, borderline personality disorder, schizophrenia, substance abuse, and self-injury. It offers suggestions for recognizing suicide warning signs, and it explains the most commonly used treatments for suicidal ideation, including counseling and medications. A section on suicide loss addresses the complex grief experienced by those who are affected by a suicide death. The book concludes with a list of crisis hotlines and a directory of additional resources for further information.

How To Use This Book

This book is divided into parts and chapters. Parts focus on broad areas of interest; chapters are devoted to single topics within a part.

Part One: Suicide Facts And Statistics provides information about the occurrence of suicide in the United States and around the world among teens, adults, and people of different ethnic backgrounds. It discusses the relationship between firearms and suicide, and it explains how the stigma associated with receiving mental health services can contribute to suicide risk by making people less likely to seek appropriate care. The part concludes with statistics and facts on suicide among LGBT youth.

Part Two: Mental Health Disorders And Life-Threatening Behaviors Linked To Suicide Risk discusses the types of mental illness that have the highest statistical links to suicide risk, including depression, bipolar disorder, anxiety disorders, border-line personality disorder, and schizophrenia. Alcohol and drug abuse, which are second only to depression and other mood disorders as the most frequent risk factors for suicide, are also addressed, and several chapters offer facts about other related concerns, including abusive relationships, bullying, self-injury, and eating disorders.

Part Three: Recognizing And Treating Suicidal Ideation offers tips about identifying the types of suicidal thoughts and behaviors, the warning signs that may precede a suicide attempt, and the psychological and medical treatments that are available for dealing with suicidal thoughts. Information is also provided about recovering from a suicide attempt and planning for a hopeful future.

Part Four: When Someone You Know Dies From Suicide explains the facets of grief often experienced by people left behind after a suicide. It offers suggestions for working through the grieving process and for supporting others who are grieving.

Part Five: Preventing Suicide discusses important components of mental health and offers practical suggestions for helping someone who may be depressed or experiencing suicidal thoughts. It discusses suicide as a preventable problem and identifies ways in which suicidal behaviors can be reduced, and provides suggestions for helping a suicidal person.

Part Six: If You Need More Information includes a list of crisis hotlines and a directory of organizations able to provide more information about suicide, suicide prevention, and suicide risk factors. It also includes a list of mobile apps for mental health.

Bibliographic Note

This volume contains documents and excerpts from publications issued by the following U.S. government agencies: Administration for Children and Families (ACF); Centers for Disease Control and Prevention (CDC); Indian Health Service (IHS); National Cancer Institute (NCI); National Center for Biotechnology Information (NCBI); National Criminal Justice Reference Service (NCJRS); National Heart, Lung, and Blood Institute (NHLBI); National Human Genome Research Institute (NHGRI); National Institute of Mental Health (NIMH); National Institute on Drug Abuse (NIDA); *NIH News in Health*; Office on Women's Health (OWH); Substance Abuse and Mental Health Services Administration (SAMHSA); U.S. Department of Health and Human Services (HHS); U.S. Department of Veterans Affairs (VA); U.S. House of Representatives; and Youth.gov.

In addition, this volume contains copyrighted document from the following organization:

The Brady Center to Prevent Gun Violence

It may also contain original material produced by Omnigraphics and reviewed by medical consultants.

The photograph on the front cover is © Laflor/iStock.

Medical Review

Omnigraphics contracts with a team of qualified, senior medical professionals who serve as medical consultants for the *Teen Health Series*. As necessary, medical consultants review reprinted and originally written material for currency and accuracy. Citations including the phrase, Reviewed (month, year)" indicate material reviewed by this team. Medical consultation services are provided to the *Teen Health Series* editors by:

Dr. Senthil Selvan, MBBS, DCH, MD
Dr. K. Sivanandham, MBBS, DCH, MS (Research), PhD

About The *Teen Health Series*

At the request of librarians serving today's young adults, the *Teen Health Series* was developed as a specially focused set of volumes within Omnigraphics' *Health Reference Series*. Each volume deals comprehensively with a topic selected according to the needs and interests of people in middle school and high school. Teens seeking preventive guidance, information about disease warning signs, medical statistics, and risk factors for health problems will find answers to their questions in the *Teen Health Series*. The *Series*, however, is not intended to serve as a tool for diagnosing illness, in prescribing treatments, or as a substitute for the physician/patient relationship. All people concerned about medical symptoms or the possibility of disease are encouraged to seek professional care from an appropriate healthcare provider.

If there is a topic you would like to see addressed in a future volume of the *Teen Health Series*, please write to:

Editor
Teen Health Series
Omnigraphics
615 Griswold, Ste. 901
Detroit, MI 48226

A Note About Spelling And Style

Teen Health Series editors use *Stedman's Medical Dictionary* as an authority for questions related to the spelling of medical terms and the *Chicago Manual of Style* for questions related to grammatical structures, punctuation, and other editorial concerns. Consistent adherence is not always possible, however, because the individual volumes within the *Series* include many documents from a wide variety of different producers and copyright holders, and the editor's primary goal is to present material from each source as accurately as is possible following the terms specified by each document's producer. This sometimes means that information in different chapters or sections may follow other guidelines and alternate spelling authorities.

Part One
Suicide Facts And Statistics

Chapter 1
Suicide In The United States

Suicide does not discriminate. People of all genders, ages, and ethnicities can be at risk for suicide. But people most at risk tend to share certain characteristics. The main risk factors for suicide are:

- depression, other mental disorders, or substance abuse disorder

- a prior suicide attempt

- family history of a mental disorder or substance abuse

- family history of suicide

- family violence, including physical or sexual abuse

- having guns or other firearms in the home

- incarceration, being in prison or jail

- being exposed to others' suicidal behavior, such as that of family members, peers, or media figures

The risk for suicidal behavior is complex. Research suggests that people who attempt suicide differ from others in many aspects of how they think, react to events, and make decisions. There are differences in aspects of memory, attention, planning, and emotion, for example. These differences often occur along with disorders like depression, substance use, anxiety, and psychosis. Sometimes suicidal behavior is triggered by events such as personal loss or violence. In order to be able to detect those at risk and prevent suicide, it is crucial that we understand the role of both long-term factors—such as experiences in childhood—and more immediate

About This Chapter: This chapter includes text excerpted from "Suicide In America: Frequently Asked Questions (2015)," National Institute of Mental Health (NIMH), April 2015.

It's A Fact!!

- Suicide was the tenth leading cause of death for all ages in 2013.
- There were 41,149 suicides in 2013 in the United States—a rate of 12.6 per 100,000 is equal to 113 suicides each day or one every 13 minutes.
- Based on data about suicides in 16 National Violent Death Reporting System states in 2010, 33.4 percent of suicide decedents tested positive for alcohol, 23.8 percent for anti-depressants, and 20.0 percent for opiates, including heroin and prescription pain killers.
- Suicide results in an estimated $51 billion in combined medical and work loss costs.

(Source: "Suicide: Facts At A Glance," Centers for Disease Control and Prevention (CDC).)

factors like mental health and recent life events. Researchers are also looking at how genes can either increase risk or make someone more resilient to loss and hardships.

Many people have some of these risk factors but do not attempt suicide.

Suicide is not a normal response to stress. It is, however, a sign of extreme distress, not a harmless bid for attention.

Nonfatal Suicidal Thoughts And Behavior

Among students in grades 9–12 in the United States during 2013:

- 17.0 percent of students seriously considered attempting suicide in the previous 12 months (22.4 percent of females and 11.6 percent of males).
- 13.6 percent of students made a plan about how they would attempt suicide in the previous 12 months (16.9 percent of females and 10.3 percent of males).
- 8.0 percent of students attempted suicide one or more times in the previous 12 months (10.6 percent of females and 5.4 percent of males).
- 2.7 percent of students made a suicide attempt that resulted in an injury, poisoning, or an overdose that required medical attention (3.6 percent of females and 1.8 percent of males).

(Source: "Suicide: Facts At A Glance," Centers for Disease Control and Prevention (CDC).)

Suicide In America: Frequently Asked Questions
What About Gender?

Men are more likely to die by suicide than women, but women are more likely to attempt suicide. Men are more likely to use deadlier methods, such as firearms or suffocation. Women are more likely than men to attempt suicide by poisoning.

A Quick Look At The Numbers

- Males take their own lives at nearly four times the rate of females and represent 77.9 percent of all suicides.
- Females are more likely than males to have suicidal thoughts.
- Suicide is the seventh leading cause of death for males and the fourteenth leading cause for females.
- Firearms are the most commonly used method of suicide among males (56.9%).
- Poisoning is the most common method of suicide for females (34.8%).

(Source: "Suicide: Facts At A Glance," Centers for Disease Control and Prevention (CDC).)

What About Children?

Children and young people are at risk for suicide. Suicide is the second leading cause of death for young people ages 15 to 34.

What About Older Adults?

Older adults are at risk for suicide, too. While older adults were the demographic group with the highest suicide rates for decades, suicide rates for middle-aged adults has increased to comparable levels (ages 24–62). Among those age 65+, white males comprise over 80 percent of all late-life suicides.

What About Different Ethnic Groups?

Among ethnicities, American Indians and Alaska Natives (AI/AN) tend to have the highest rate of suicides, followed by non-Hispanic Whites. Hispanics, African Americans, and Asian/Pacific Islanders each have suicide rates that are about half their White and AI/AN counterparts.

Numbers To Note

- Suicide is the eighth leading cause of death among American Indians / Alaska Natives across all ages.
- Among American Indians / Alaska Natives aged 10 to 34 years, suicide is the second leading cause of death.
- The suicide rate among American Indian / Alaska Native adolescents and young adults ages 15 to 34 (19.5 per 100,000) is 1.5 times higher than the national average for that age group (12.9 per 100,000).

- The percentages of adults aged 18 or older having suicidal thoughts in the previous 12 months were 2.9 percent among blacks, 3.3 percent among Asians, 3.6 percent among Hispanics, 4.1 percent among whites, 4.6 percent among Native Hawaiians / Other Pacific Islanders, 4.8 percent among American Indians /Alaska Natives, and 7.9 percent among adults reporting two or more races.

- Among Hispanic students in grades 9–12, the prevalence of having seriously considered attempting suicide (18.9%), having made a plan about how they would attempt suicide (15.7%), having attempted suicide (11.3%), and having made a suicide attempt that resulted in an injury, poisoning, or overdose that required medical attention (4.1%) was consistently higher than white and black students.

(Source: "Suicide: Facts At A Glance," Centers for Disease Control and Prevention (CDC).)

Chapter 2
Statistics On Suicide In The United States

Suicide is a major public health concern. Suicide is among the leading causes of death in the United States. Based on recent nationwide surveys, suicide in some populations is on the rise.

- Suicide is defined as death caused by self-directed injurious behavior with intent to die as a result of the behavior.

- A suicide attempt is a non-fatal, self-directed, potentially injurious behavior with intent to die as a result of the behavior. A suicide attempt might not result in injury.

- Suicidal ideation refers to thinking about, considering, or planning suicide.

Suicide Is A Leading Cause Of Death In The United States

According to the Centers for Disease Control and Prevention (CDC), in 2014:

- Suicide was the tenth leading cause of death overall in the United States, claiming the lives of more than 42,000 people.

- Suicide was the second leading cause of death among individuals between the ages of 10 and 34.

- There were more than twice as many suicides (42,773) in the United States as there were homicides (15,809).

About This Chapter: This chapter includes text excerpted from "Suicide," National Institute of Mental Health (NIMH), September 4, 2016.

Suicide Rates

Trends Over Time

- Suicide rate is based on the number of people who have died by suicide per 100,000 populations. Because changes in population size are taken into account, rates allow for comparisons from one year to the next.

- Figure 2.1 shows the age-adjusted suicide rates in the United States for each year from 1999 through 2014 for the total population, and for males and females presented separately.

  - Over the past 15 years, the total suicide rate has increased 24 percent from 10.5 to 13.0 per 100,000.

  - The suicide rate among males has remained approximately four times higher (20.7 per 100,000 in 2014) than among females (5.8 per 100,000 in 2014).

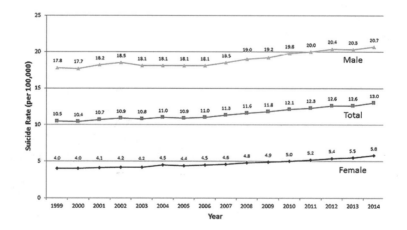

Figure 2.1. Age-Adjusted Suicide Rates In The United States (1999–2014)

Demographics

- Because suicide rates take population size into account, they can be a useful tool for understanding the relative proportion of people affected within different demographic groups.

- Figure 2.2 shows the rates of suicide within sex and age categories in 2014.

- Among females, the suicide rate was highest for those aged 45–64 (9.8 per 100,000).

- Among males, the suicide rate was highest for those aged 75 and over (38.8 per 100,000).

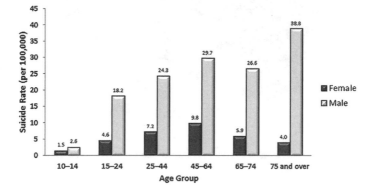

Figure 2.2. Suicide Rates By Age In The United States (2014)

- Figure 2.3 shows the rates of suicide within race/ethnicity groups in 2014. The rates of suicide were highest for males (27.4 per 100,000) and females (8.7 per 100,000) in the American Indian / Alaska Native group, followed by males (25.8 per 100,000) and females (7.5 per 100,000) in the White / non-Hispanic group.

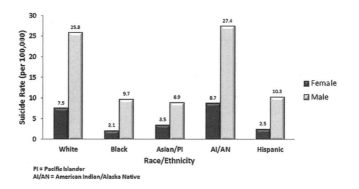

Figure 2.3. Suicide Rates By Race/Ethnicity In The United States (2014)

Suicide Rates By State

- Suicide rates are not the same from state to state. Based on data from the CDC, Figure 2.4 shows a map of the United States with each state's average suicide rate from 2004 to 2010 indicated by color.

9

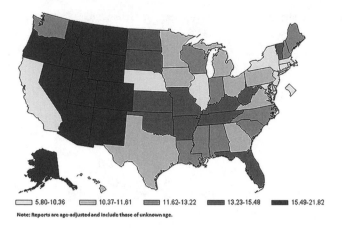

5.80-10.36   10.37-11.61   11.62-13.22   13.23-15.48   15.49-21.82

Note: Reports are age-adjusted and include those of unknown age.

Figure 2.4. Suicide Rates In The United States (By State; Per 100,000; Average 2004–2010)

Suicide Method

Number Of Suicide Deaths By Method

- Table 2.1 includes information on the total number of suicides for the most common methods.

- In 2014, firearms were the most common method used in suicide deaths in the United States, accounting for almost half of all suicide deaths (21,334).

Table 2.1. Number Of Suicide Deaths By Method

Suicide Method	Number Of Deaths (2014)
Total	42,773
Firearm	21,334
Suffocation	11,407
Poisoning	6,808
Other	3,224

Percent Of Suicide Deaths By Method

- Figure 2.5 shows the percentages of suicide deaths by method among males and females.

- Poisoning was the most common method of suicide among females in 2014, accounting for about one-third (34.1%) of all female suicides.

- More than half of male suicides (55.4%) in 2014 were firearm-related.

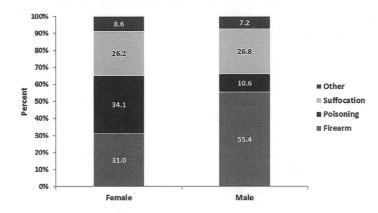

Figure 2.5. Suicide Deaths By Method In The United States (2014)

Cost Of Suicide Deaths

- In addition to the emotional loss associated with suicide, there is also an economic loss as the burden of suicide falls most heavily on adults of working age.

- Figure 2.6 shows the medical and work-loss costs of fatal injury by intent in the United States in 2013, reported by the CDC.

- Suicide accounted for $50.8 billion (24%) of the fatal injury cost.

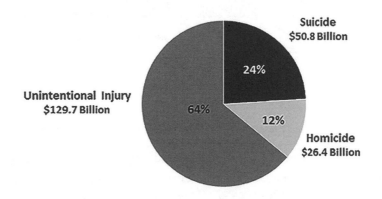

Figure 2.6. Medical And Work-Loss Costs Of Fatal Injury By Intent In The United States (2013)

11

Suicidal Thoughts And Behaviors Among U.S. Adults

- In Figure 2.7, data from the 2014 National Survey on Drug Use and Health (NSDUH) by the Substance Abuse and Mental Health Services Administration (SAMHSA) show that 3.9 percent of adults age 18 and older in the United States had thoughts about suicide in the past year.

- The percentage of adults having serious thoughts of suicide was highest among adults aged 18–25 (7.5%).

- The prevalence of suicidal thoughts was highest among adults reporting two or more races (8.3%).

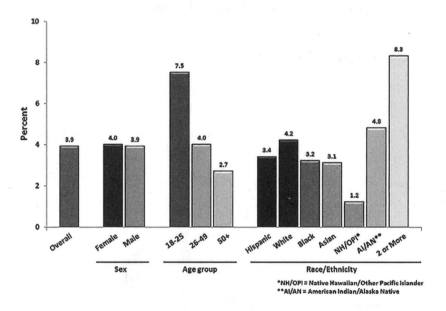

Figure 2.7. Past Year Prevalence Of Suicidal Thoughts Among U.S. Adults (2014)

- Figure 2.8 shows that in 2014, 9.4 million adults aged 18 or older reported having serious thoughts about trying to kill themselves, and 1.1 million adults aged 18 or older attempted suicide during the past year. Among those adults who attempted suicide, 0.9 million also reported making suicide plans.

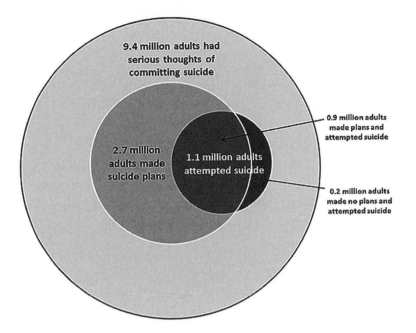

Figure 2.8. Past Year Suicidal Thoughts And Behaviors Among U.S. Adults (2014)

Chapter 3
Teen Suicide Statistics

Youth Suicide

Suicide (i.e., taking one's own life) is a serious public health problem that affects even young people. For youth between the ages of 10 and 24, suicide is the third leading cause of death. It results in approximately 4600 lives lost each year. The top three methods used in suicides of young people include firearm (45%), suffocation (40%), and poisoning (8%).

Deaths from youth suicide are only part of the problem. More young people survive suicide attempts than actually die. A nationwide survey of youth in grades 9–12 in public and private schools in the United States found that 16 percent of students reported seriously considering suicide, 13 percent reported creating a plan, and 8 percent reporting trying to take their own life in the 12 months preceding the survey. Each year, approximately 157,000 youth between the ages of 10 and 24 receive medical care for self-inflicted injuries at Emergency Departments across the United States.

Suicide affects all youth, but some groups are at higher risk than others. Boys are more likely than girls to die from suicide. Of the reported suicides in the 10 to 24 age group, 81 percent of the deaths were males and 19 percent were females. Girls, however, are more likely to report attempting suicide than boys. Cultural variations in suicide rates also exist, with Native American / Alaskan Native youth having the highest rates of suicide-related fatalities. A nationwide survey of youth in grades 9–12 in public and private schools in the United States found Hispanic youth were more likely to report attempting suicide than their black and white, non-Hispanic peers.

About This Chapter: This chapter includes text excerpted from "Suicide Prevention," Centers for Disease Control and Prevention (CDC), March 10, 2015.

Several factors can put a young person at risk for suicide. However, having these risk factors does not always mean that suicide will occur.

Risk Factors

- History of previous suicide attempts

- Family history of suicide

- History of depression or other mental illness

- Alcohol or drug abuse

- Stressful life event or loss

- Easy access to lethal methods

- Exposure to the suicidal behavior of others

- Incarceration

Most people are uncomfortable with the topic of suicide. Too often, victims are blamed, and their families and friends are left stigmatized. As a result, people do not communicate openly about suicide. Thus an important public health problem is left shrouded in secrecy, which limits the amount of information available to those working to prevent suicide.

The good news is that research over the last several decades has uncovered a wealth of information on the causes of suicide and on prevention strategies. Additionally, Centers for Disease Control and Prevention (CDC) is working to monitor the problem and develop programs to prevent youth suicide.

It's A Fact!!

Among persons aged 10–24 years, suicide rates are higher in males than in females. Suicide rates by suffocation (including hanging) have been increasing among females in this age group since the early 1990s.

These results highlight the increased use of suffocation as a method of suicide among young persons. Professionals who work with young persons and their families need to be aware of the trend in this highly lethal method when asking about suicide plans and when working to reduce suicide risk. These results also underscore the importance of early prevention of suicidal behavior and effective intervention for youth and young adults at greater risk for suicide.

Chapter 4
Teen Suicide: A Global Perspective

Suicide accounts for an estimated 800,000 deaths each year, according to the World Health Organization (WHO), making it the fifth-leading cause of death worldwide. Many experts believe the true number may be higher because some deaths are unreported or misclassified due to the sensitive nature of suicide. The scope of the problem appears even larger when you consider that there are many unsuccessful suicide attempts for each completed suicide. Since every suicide has tragic, long-lasting consequences for that person's family and community, finding ways to prevent suicide is clearly an issue of global concern.

> **Did You Know...**
> According to the WHO, a person dies by suicide somewhere in the world every 40 seconds.

Suicide affects people of all nationalities, genders, and ages. It occurs in every country in the world, regardless of its level of wealth or economic development. WHO researchers found that 75 percent of global suicides occurred in low- and middle-income countries (LMIC) in 2012. This figure is deceiving, however, because such a large proportion of the world's population lives in LMIC. In fact, the suicide rate of 11.2 per 100,000 people in LMIC was lower than the rate of 12.7 per 100,000 people found in high-income countries. A country's location or region seems to make little difference in the prevalence of suicide. Countries from all parts of the world appear near both the top and bottom of the global ranking of all nations by suicide rate.

"Teen Suicide: A Global Perspective," © 2017 Omnigraphics. Reviewed January 2017.

Men are more likely to die by suicide than women. This trend is most pronounced in high-income countries, where an average of 3.5 men committed suicide for every woman who did so in 2012. In LMIC the male-to-female ratio was much lower, at 1.6 men for every woman. In most regions of the world, suicide is most common among elderly people over the age of 70. But suicide claims many lives among younger people between the ages of 15 and 29, as well. In fact, suicide accounts for 8.5 percent of all deaths in this age group, compared to 4.1 percent of all deaths among middle-aged people between 30 and 49. This makes suicide the second-leading cause of death (after accidents) for younger people worldwide.

Suicide Among Teens

Globally, the highest rates of teen suicide can be found in the regions of Southeast Asia and Eastern Europe. Teenage boys have higher suicide rates than teenage girls in most countries (with the exception of China and India). Teenagers who are members of native or indigenous ethnic minority groups face a significantly higher risk of suicide than teens who are members of the majority population.

In the United States, suicide is second only to accidents as the leading cause of death among 15- to 19-year-olds. From 1999 to 2014, the teen suicide rate in the United States rose from 8.0 to 8.7 per 100,000 people. Researchers believe that the number of suicide attempts remained relatively stable during this period, however, and blame the increase on teens using more lethal methods of suicide. The suicide rate among teens who live in rural areas of the United States, at 11.9 deaths per 100,000, is nearly twice the rate of 6.5 among teens who live in urban areas. Teens in rural areas frequently experience poverty and social isolation, while they are less likely to have access to mental healthcare services.

Risk Factors For Suicide

There are many different risk factors that can contribute to suicidal behavior. On an individual level, the main drivers of suicide include mental disorders, depression, and substance abuse. A family history of suicide and previous suicide attempts are also major risk factors. Although these factors affect individuals worldwide, their impact is greatest in countries where people feel unable to seek help because of the social stigma attached to mental health issues and suicide.

Many suicides occur during moments of emotional crisis, when people feel overwhelmed and unable to cope with sources of stress in their daily lives. For teenagers, peer pressure, bullying, social isolation, and relationship troubles are common factors that contribute to suicidal behavior. Suicide rates are highest worldwide among young people in vulnerable groups that are likely to experience discrimination or marginalization, such as refugees and migrants, racial and ethnic minorities, and lesbian, gay, bisexual, and transgender (LGBT) persons.

Among middle-aged people, financial problems are a common driver of suicidal behavior. Men in this age group, in particular, feel pressure to provide for their families and achieve financial stability. Among elderly people, health-related issues frequently contribute to suicidal behavior. Those who face chronic pain and illness sometimes view suicide as a way to avoid losing their independence or becoming a burden to their families.

Some of the risk factors for suicide occur on a larger, national scale. Countries that experience wars, ethnic conflicts, and violence often have much higher suicide rates than countries that are more stable. Natural disasters, such as earthquakes or hurricanes, are also associated with increases in suicide rates. People who experience trauma, loss, or displacement due to these events face high levels of stress that make them more vulnerable to suicidal behavior.

Inappropriate media reporting may also contribute to the problem by sensationalizing suicide and making it seem like an acceptable option. In 1978, at the Jonestown settlement in the South American nation of Guyana, a cult leader named Jim Jones ordered his followers to drink poison. The mass suicide of 900 people received huge amounts of media coverage. From that time onward, Guyana's relatively low suicide rate increased rapidly until it reached the highest level in the Western Hemisphere. Researchers cited the publicity surrounding the Jonestown incident as a major factor in increasing the awareness and prevalence of suicide among Guyana's youth. Teens tend to be most susceptible to the phenomenon of "copycat" suicides.

Methods Of Suicide

The most common means of suicide worldwide is self-poisoning with pesticides, which accounts for about one-third of global suicides. People who live in rural, agricultural areas in LMIC often have easy access to these deadly chemicals. Other common means include hanging and firearms. The methods used vary greatly, however, depending on the country and age group. Since many suicides result from spur-of-the-moment, impulsive decisions, people tend to choose the method that is most available to them.

Prevention Of Suicide

Suicide prevention requires a comprehensive, coordinated approach by multiple sectors of government and society, including healthcare, education, law, business, and the media. In many countries, however, suicide prevention is not considered an important topic of research or discussion. Without accurate data collection and statistics, many people are not aware of the extent of the problem. In addition, the stigma surrounding mental health and suicide in some countries makes people reluctant to discuss the issue or seek help. As a result, only 28 countries of the nearly 200 countries in the world have a national suicide prevention strategy in place.

The WHO is committed to raising public awareness of suicide worldwide and encouraging countries to take positive action to prevent it. Under the WHO Mental Health Action Plan, released in 2013, member countries agreed to work toward reducing the global suicide rate by 10 percent by 2020. Strategies for preventing suicide address the problem at three main levels: the universal or national level; the selective or population subgroup level; and the individual level.

At the national level, WHO efforts are aimed at improving access to mental healthcare, creating policies to reduce substance abuse, and promoting economic development and anti-poverty programs. Other strategies at the national level may involve encouraging responsible media reporting or restricting access to the means of suicide, such as firearms or pesticides. This approach produced results in the United Kingdom, where self-poisoning with carbon monoxide gas from coal-burning furnaces once accounted for half of all suicides. After the government phased out coal in favor of natural gas as a heating source in the 1960s, the national suicide rate fell by one-third permanently.

Selective suicide prevention strategies target vulnerable population groups within a country or region. Such strategies might take steps to increase community support for people affected by wars or natural disasters, or they might provide education to reduce discrimination against racial and ethnic minorities.

At the individual level, suicide prevention strategies aim to improve early identification and treatment of mental disorders, substance abuse issues, emotional distress, and chronic pain. Tactics might include training healthcare workers to recognize suicidal behavior, providing follow-up treatment for people who attempt suicide, and offering positive coping methods and community support.

A vital factor in all types of suicide prevention efforts is information. Researchers must have access to high-quality data from hospitals, law enforcement, and surveys in order to identify the patterns, characteristics, and methods of suicide in each country or part of the world. This data enables researchers to track changes in suicide rates and understand the factors driving them. In this way, they can design timely, comprehensive interventions to address the underlying problems and effectively prevent suicides.

References

1. Goldberg, Sara. "No Easy Way Out: An Overview Of International Trends In Suicide," GenRe, April 2014.

2. McLoughlin, A. B., M. S. Gould, and K. M. Malone. "Global Trends In Teenage Suicide: 2003–2014," QJM: An International Journal of Medicine, January 2015, pp. 765–780.

3. "Preventing Suicide: A Global Imperative," World Health Organization (WHO), 2014.

4. "Suicide Fact Sheet," World Health Organization (WHO), September 2016.

5. "Suicide Rates By Country," World Atlas, 2016.

Chapter 5
Suicide In Older Adults

Suicide is an important public health problem in the United States and a tragedy for all involved—families, friends, neighbors, colleagues, and communities. In 2013, suicide was the 10th leading cause of death in the United States overall. Among people aged 15 to 54, suicide ranked even higher as a cause of death.

However, research suggests that there are many more attempted suicides than there are deaths from suicide. People also are likely to have thought about suicide before actually attempting suicide.

(Source: "Suicidal Thoughts And Behavior Among Adults: Results From The 2014 National Survey On Drug Use And Health," Substance Abuse and Mental Health Services Administration (SAMHSA).)

9.4 Million American Adults Had Serious Thoughts Of Suicide In 2014

A report by the Substance Abuse and Mental Health Services Administration (SAMHSA) reveals that in 2014, 3.9 percent of American adults aged 18 and older thought seriously about killing themselves during the past 12 months. During this same period, 1.1 percent of adults made suicide plans, and 0.5 percent of adults made non-fatal attempts at suicide.

About This Chapter: Text under the heading "9.4 Million American Adults Had Serious Thoughts Of Suicide In 2014" is excerpted from "9.4 Million American Adults Had Serious Thoughts Of Suicide In 2014," Substance Abuse and Mental Health Services Administration (SAMHSA), September 10, 2015; Text under the heading "Preventing Suicide Among Older Adults" is excerpted from "Preventing Suicide Among Seniors," Substance Abuse and Mental Health Services Administration (SAMHSA), February 2, 2016.

23

Adults with substance use disorders or major depressive episodes had higher rates of serious suicide thought and behaviors.

More than 40,000 people in the United States die from suicide annually, according to the Centers for Disease Control and Prevention (CDC)—making suicide the 10th leading cause of death among people aged 15 to 54.

The SAMHSA report shows that the percentage of adults who had serious thoughts of attempting suicide over the past 12 months has remained relatively stable since SAMHSA started tracking this issue in 2008.

About one third of adults who had serious thoughts of suicide in the past year also made suicide plans. One in nine adults who had serious thoughts of suicide in the past year made a non-lethal suicide attempt.

The report shows some differences in the levels of suicidal thoughts and behaviors among certain groups. For example, 11.9 percent of adults with a substance use disorder in the past 12 months had serious thoughts of suicide, 3.9 percent of these adults made suicide plans and 2.1 percent of these adults made non-fatal attempts at suicide.

Similarly, rates of suicidal thoughts and behaviors were higher among adults who experienced a major depressive episode in the past 12 months. Nearly one third of these adults (29.5 percent) have serious thoughts of suicide, 9.7 percent made suicide plans and 3.4 percent made non-fatal attempts at suicide.

The report also shows that only about half (51.4 percent) of adults who had serious thoughts of suicide in the past 12 month had received mental health services.

Preventing Suicide Among Older Adults

More than 7,000 people age 65 or older died by suicide in 2013, according to statistics from the CDC—a figure that places the suicide rate among older adults higher than the general population. Suicide rates are particularly high among older men—higher than among any other group in the United States. And these figures do not include those who have made suicide attempts or who suffer from the emotional pain of suicidal thoughts.

Older adults, like their younger cohorts, are more likely to have suicidal thoughts if they have depression and mood disorders or substance use problems.

But unlike younger people, they are also more likely to be dealing with other issues that can produce suicidal thoughts, including medical conditions and pain that affect function and autonomy. Many older adults also face social isolation that sometimes results from the loss of a loved one, the inability to get around without help, or the feeling that they are a burden to others.

In the case of those who are living alone, it's often difficult to spot the warning signs that accompany suicide. Making matters worse, those in older generations are often less likely to seek out help.

What You Can Do

If you work with older adults and someone you know may be experiencing risk factors for suicide:

- Talk with the person in a caring, nonjudgmental way.

- Encourage the person to attend wellness sessions or classes offered by your senior center.

- Connect the person to supportive services available from the senior center (e.g., Meals on Wheels programs, assistance with financial planning).

- Connect the person to sources of counseling or other forms of support.

Suicide Risk And Risk Of Death Among Recent Veterans

A study of Veterans serving during the Iraq and Afghanistan wars between 2001–2007 found that both deployed and non-deployed Veterans had a significantly higher suicide risk compared to the U.S. general population, but a lower risk of death from other causes combined. Also, deployed Veterans showed a lower risk of suicide compared to non-deployed Veterans. Veterans were followed through the end of 2009.

Risk comparison among Veterans serving during the Iraq and Afghanistan wars between 2001–2007:

- Deployed Veterans had a 41 percent higher suicide risk compared to the general U.S. population.
- Non-deployed Veterans had a 61 percent higher suicide risk compared to the general U.S. population.

Deaths among Veterans serving during the Iraq and Afghanistan wars between 2001–2007 (Veterans were followed through the end of 2009):

- Deployed: 317,581 total Veterans, 1,650 total deaths. 21.3% death by suicide.
- Non-deployed: 964,493 total Veterans, 7,703 total deaths. 19.7% death by suicide.
- Deployed Veterans showed a lower risk of suicide compared to non-deployed Veterans.
- Female Veteran suicide rates were about a third of the suicide rate of male Veterans.

- Suicide rate of female Veterans: 11.2 out of 100,000 Veterans.
- Suicide rate of male Veterans: 33.4 out of 100,000 Veterans.

The increased risk of suicide among female Veterans when compared to the U.S. female population was higher than that observed when male Veterans were compared to the U.S. male population, regardless of deployment status.

Suicides by gender and deployment:

- Deployed suicides: 15 suicides among females, 336 suicides among males.
- Non-deployed suicides: 109 suicides among females, 1,408 suicides among males.

Regardless of deployment status, the suicide risk was higher among younger, male, white, unmarried, enlisted, and Army/Marine Veterans; however, predictors of suicide were similar between male and female Veterans.

Suicide rate by year since discharge by deployment status of Veterans (rate calculated per 100,000 person years at risk):

- Within 3 years since discharge, 33.1 suicide rate by non-deployed Veterans, 29.7 suicide rate by deployed Veterans.
- Within 6 years since discharge, 27.3 suicide rate by non-deployed Veterans, 24.7 suicide rate by deployed Veterans.
- Within 9 years since discharge, 25.6 suicide rate by non-deployed Veterans, 26.1 suicide rate by deployed Veterans.

The rate of suicide was greatest within 3 years after leaving service.

(Source: "Suicide Risk And Risk Of Death Among Recent Veterans," Veterans Health Administration (VHA), U.S. Department of Veterans Affairs (VA).)

Chapter 6
Culture Plays A Role In Adolescent Suicide

Knowledge of the risk factors for suicidal behavior in youth has burgeoned during the past 20 years. Converging evidence points to psychiatric or mental disorders as well as a past history of suicidal behavior as the strongest predictors of suicidal behavior and death by suicide. However, the role of social and cultural factors is less clear and remains a topic of theoretical and practical interest. Given that social contextual factors can significantly impact well-being, they might also serve as predictors of suicidal behavior and a basis for formulating preventive measures.

The present review focuses on recent developments in our understanding of the social and cultural aspects of youth suicide and suicidal behavior and their implications for prevention. Suicidal behavior is a set of noncontinuous and heterogeneous spectra of behaviors, such that suicidal ideation, suicidal threats, gestures, self-cutting, low lethal suicide attempts, interrupted suicide attempts, near-fatal suicide attempts, and actual suicide may or may not be related to each other, depending on the context in which they are studied.

Social Theories Of Suicide

According to several major theorists in the field of suicidology, social and cultural variables need to be taken into account in the understanding of suicide. Durkheim, considered the founder of empirical research in sociology and suicidology, hypothesized in his 1897 book *Suicide* that suicide rates vary negatively with the level of social integration (conceptualized as the opposite of anomia, isolation and egoism) of individual groups. He also highlighted the roles of religious integration and varying family circumstances. Since then many biosocial

About This Chapter: This chapter includes text excerpted from "Social Aspects Of Suicidal Behavior And Prevention In Early Life: A Review," National Center for Biotechnology Information (NCBI), November 3, 2016.

models of self-harmful behavior have incorporated family processes and social support networks and support the promotion of social cohesion and identification with societal values in the enhancement of mental health in general and the prevention of suicide in particular. In adolescents, in whom identity is a vital element of well-being, this could be accomplished through participation in youth movements, social clubs, sports activities, and national service.

Epidemiology: Cultural And Ethnic Issues

Adolescent suicidal behaviors are widespread and produce a significant burden on healthcare systems. In the United States, suicide is the fourth most common cause of death among 10–14-year-olds, and the third most common cause of death among 15–24-year-olds. The epidemiology of adolescent suicide has shown striking changes over the last 100 years, with a steady decline in recent decades. One of the factors suggested to explain this trend is the growing use of antidepressants, especially selective serotonin reuptake inhibitors, in the adolescent population.

The prevalence of suicidal behaviors varies significantly across countries, cultures, and racial/ethnic groups worldwide. Even within the same country, there are considerable differences among populations. In the United States, for example, adolescents of Indian/Alaskan descent have the highest rates of fatal suicidal behavior of all ethnic groups, and Latino and Caucasian youth have the highest rates of ideation and deliberate self-harm (DSH). Similarly, extremely high rates of suicide have been recorded for adolescents among the Inuit populations in Canada and the Ethiopian population in Israel, which share a pattern of a failure of a traditional culture to integrate with modern Western culture.

Suicide is the second leading cause of death among American Indian and Alaska Native youth ages 8 to 24. Furthermore, American Indian and Alaska Native high school students report higher rates of suicidal behaviors (serious thoughts of suicide, making suicide plans, attempting suicide, and getting medical attention for a suicide attempt) than the general population of U.S. high school students.

Of students in grades 9 to 12, significantly more Hispanic/Latina female students (13.5%) reported attempting suicide in the last year as compared to Black, non-Hispanic female students (8.8%) and White, non-Hispanic female students (7.9%). One national study found that perceived caring from teachers was associated with a decreased risk of suicide attempts by Latina adolescents.

(Source: "Cultural Awareness And Competency Around Suicide Prevention," Substance Abuse and Mental Health Services Administration (SAMHSA).)

The large majority of suicides (90.5%) occur among Caucasian Americans. However, the rate for black adolescent males has been rising significantly and now approximates that of European Americans. Interestingly, only about half of all black adolescent suicide attempters report ever having received a diagnosis of a mental disorder (by accepted criteria); this rate is much lower than rates reported in previous studies of adolescents in general. This finding highlights the importance of moving beyond the study of mental disorders to a broader range of factors to improve our understanding of how suicidal behavior develops.

Another recent epidemiological finding is the variation in the characteristics of youth suicide between Asian and Western countries. In rural China, southern India, Sri Lanka and Singapore, the gender differences for suicide are reversed from those in the West, with young women being at higher risk for suicide than young men; the mode of suicide attempts differs accordingly, consisting mostly of the impulsive use of pesticides. Unlike Western suicidal youth, female attempters in China do not appear to have major mental illnesses. These data have important theoretical and preventive implications.

Risk Factors For Suicidal Behavior

Major established risk factors for suicide in youth include a previous suicide attempt, availability of lethal means, and family discord. However, most of the studies focused on Caucasian youth, and less is known about the suicidal behavior of ethnic minorities.

Some of the important social risk factors underlying adolescent suicidal behavior:

Gender

In Western countries, the rates of suicide across ethnicities are higher in adolescent boys than adolescent girls (ratio of 5:1), whereas the rates of suicidal ideation and attempted suicide are higher in girls (ratio of 3:1). Explanations for the higher suicide rate in boys include higher suicidal intent, use of more violent methods, higher prevalence of antisocial disorder and substance abuse, and greater vulnerability to stressors, such as legal difficulties, financial problems, and interpersonal loss. Boys may also have more difficulties in asking for help and communicating their distress. The gender gap in DSH is most pronounced among youths of Caucasian American descent and least pronounced among American Indians. The gender gap in suicide mortality has been widening in recent decades, especially in some ethnic minority groups in the United States, mostly because of the increase in suicide among ethnic minority boys accompanied by stable suicide mortality rates among girls of all ethnic groups.

A key issue in adolescent suicidal behavior is the different impact of certain risk factors by gender. Some risk factors lead to different suicidal behaviors (fatal/nonfatal) in boys and girls, and others are associated with suicidal behavior specifically in girls but not boys or vice versa. For example, depression appears to be a better predictor of suicidal behavior in European American girls than boys, whereas alcohol abuse, substance abuse, and conduct disorders appear to be stronger correlates of suicidal behavior in European American boys than girls. In the United States, sexual abuse is increasingly being recognized as a factor in girls' DSH. Conflict with parents seems to create a unique vulnerability of girls to DSH. Others found that social isolation from peers and intransitive friendships significantly increase the odds of suicidal ideation in girls, and being part of a tightly networked school community (high relative density of friendship ties) is protective against suicide attempts in boys. Thus, social network variables are relevant to suicidality in different ways in boys and girls.

Accordingly, there may be preventive methods that are more suitable for one gender than the other. As mentioned, in Western cultures, adolescent males often find it difficult to seek help owing to social norms. Therefore, encouraging adolescent boys to communicate distress before it is too late should be a cornerstone of school and youth suicide preventive programs. This could be especially useful for young military conscripts. By contrast, girls should be encouraged to adopt more constructive coping mechanisms rather than self-injury as a means of solving interpersonal problems. Recent developments in feminist psychology, such as the practices introduced by Carol Gilligan, may be very helpful in this regard. Gilligan offers gender-based strategies for preventing psychological distress and youth violence. According to Gilligan, girls tend to suicidal behavior as a language that commands attention and respect and as an expression of a desire for relationship, while boys turn to violence as an alternative to feeling helpless and powerless. Thus, shifting the interpretation of the suicidal behavior to the relational communication of the violent intention might enable adolescent girls to verbally express their psychological distress. Moreover, strengthening healthy resistance and courage in young children (boys and girls) will prevent violence and enable these young adolescents to say what they feel and to know how to stay in a relationship with others instead of turning to suicidal behaviors.

Family Factors

Research has pointed to the importance of the family environment as a predictor of suicidal behavior among adolescents. The relevant family-related risk factors are parental psychopathology, family history of suicidal behavior, family discord, loss of a parent to death or divorce, poor quality of the parent-child relationship, and maltreatment. There is strong and convergent evidence that suicidal behavior is familial and, perhaps, genetic, and that the liability to suicidal behavior is transmitted in families independently of psychiatric disorder. Nevertheless, there may also be environmental routes of transmission, such as imitation and intergenerational family adversity. Therefore, prevention programs should be designed for early identification and treatment of potentially suicidal adolescents from dysfunctional families. Mental health professionals should be encouraged to try to improve functioning within the family of suicidal youth.

Physical And Sexual Abuse

Empirical studies overwhelmingly point to an association between childhood abuse/neglect and suicidality for both boys and girls and within different ethnic/racial groups. Exposure to physical and, especially, sexual abuse in childhood leads to a significant increase in poor mental health outcomes, including suicidal ideation and behavior, experienced at ages 16 to 25. The risk is increased if the child is sexually abused by an immediate family member or the sexual abuse is repeated over time. The greater the severity of the abuse, the higher the risk of suicide attempts. Sexually abused boys were at greater risk of suicide attempts than sexually abused girls, although both groups were at higher risk than non-abused boys and girls. Thus, all abused children and adolescents should be carefully evaluated for suicidal thoughts and behaviors, and health professionals who work with them should be trained in adolescent suicidal therapy. Several interventions have been investigated as strategies to prevent suicide in abused children, including family preservation or unification models, broad ecologically based intervention models and prevention models. One of the largest projects examined mental health interventions for children who were victims of intrafamilial physical or sexual abuse. Trauma-focused cognitive-behavioral therapy was proven effective in reducing psychological distress in these children. Moreover, it seems that better education regarding reporting suspected abuse and making it easier for children to seek help if they are being abused may also be important measures.

Change Of Residence And Socioeconomic Class

Qin et al. reported that children who frequently moved were more likely to make suicide attempts during adolescence. There was a dose-response relationship between number of moves and risk of attempted suicide. However, other studies found that residential mobility was associated with suicide attempts in adolescent females but not males, suggesting an important gender difference. More empirical research is needed in order to address this difference. Another factor is social class. Some studies show that adolescents who engage in DSH behaviors tend to be from lower socioeconomic strata, while other studies found no such association. Additionally, low levels of parental education are associated with higher adolescent suicidal risk.

Sexual Orientation

Youth who report same-sex sexual orientation are at greater risk than their peers to attempt suicide, and this risk persists even after controlling for other suicide risk factors. According to a study, gay, lesbian or bisexual adolescents who experience family rejection or a negative family reaction at their "coming out" have an eightfold greater likelihood of attempting suicide than adolescents who experience no or minimal family rejection. These findings indicate that providing the gay/lesbian adolescent community with help in resolving their identity issues is an important part of suicide prevention. Moreover, addressing the societal rejection issue seems to be an important measure in this regard.

Experiences With Violence

Negative attitudes toward lesbian, gay, and bisexual (LGB) people put these youth at increased risk for experiences with violence, compared with other students. Violence can include behaviors such as bullying, teasing, harassment, physical assault, and suicide-related behaviors.

Lesbian, gay, bisexual, transgender, and questioning (LGBTQ) youth are also at increased risk for suicidal thoughts and behaviors, suicide attempts, and suicide. A nationally representative study of adolescents in grades 7–12 found that lesbian, gay, and bisexual youth were more than twice as likely to have attempted suicide as their heterosexual peers. More studies are needed to better understand the risks for suicide among transgender youth. However, one study with 55 transgender youth found that about 25 percent reported suicide attempts.

Another survey of more than 7,000 seventh- and eighth-grade students from a large Midwestern county examined the effects of school [social] climate and homophobic bullying on lesbian, gay, bisexual, and questioning (LGBQ) youth and found that

- LGBQ youth were more likely than heterosexual youth to report high levels of bullying and substance use;
- Students who were questioning their sexual orientation reported more bullying, homophobic victimization, unexcused absences from school, drug use, feelings of depression, and suicidal behaviors than either heterosexual or LGB students;
- LGB students who did not experience homophobic teasing reported the lowest levels of depression and suicidal feelings of all student groups (heterosexual, LGB, and questioning students); and

- All students, regardless of sexual orientation, reported the lowest levels of depression, suicidal feelings, alcohol and marijuana use, and unexcused absences from school when they were
  - in a positive school climate, and
  - not experiencing homophobic teasing

(Source: "Lesbian, Gay, Bisexual, And Transgender Health: LGBT Youth," Centers for Disease Control and Prevention (CDC).)

Alcohol And Drugs

Alcohol abuse is known to be associated with an increased risk of suicidal behavior and suicide death among adolescents. A study reported that the link between heavy episodic drinking (HED) and suicide attempts is maintained even after controlling for depression. The association was strongest in the under 13-year age group and decreased with increasing age. These findings suggest that early HED may be a marker for some other factor (e.g., poor behavioral inhibition, poor decision making, cognitive precociousness) causally related to suicide attempts. Restricting alcohol sales to adolescents has already been shown to be an effective suicide-prevention measure.

Bullying

Klomek et al. showed that bullying and victimization during childhood increase the odds of a subsequent suicide attempt. However, Brent et al. found that in boys, bullying, but not victimization, was associated with suicide, but the association was not causal; rather, both bullying and suicide were both consequences of conduct disorder, a known risk factor for suicidal behavior. By contrast, in girls, victimization, but not bullying, was associated with suicide attempts, even after adjusting for conduct disorder and depression. Others reported that boys who were both bullies and victims of bullying had a higher likelihood of suicidal behavior than boys who were only victims. In girls, victims of bullying were more likely to exhibit suicidal behaviors than those who were neither bullies nor victims. Today, many youth are subject to cyberbullying through Email, cell phone texting, and Internet social sites, perpetrated by other adolescents or even adults. These findings call for strenuous efforts by school authorities to prevent bullying and the formulation of interventions to minimize its deleterious effects, particularly regarding cyberbullying.

> **What We Know And Don't Know**
>
> We don't know if bullying directly causes suicide. We know that most kids who are involved in bullying do NOT engage in suicide-related behavior. It is correct to say that involvement in bullying, along with other risk factors, can increase the chance that a young person will engage in suicide-related behaviors.
>
> We know that bullying behavior and suicide-related behavior are related. This means youth who report any involvement with bullying behavior are more likely to report suicide-related behavior than youth who do not report any involvement with bullying behavior.
>
> *(Source: "Bullying And Suicide: What's The Connection?" StopBullying.gov, U.S. Department of Health and Human Services (HHS).)*

Suicide Contagion

Social learning may be an important factor in both familial and nonfamilial transmission of suicidal behaviors. The concept of suicide contagion is based on the infective disease model and assumes that a suicidal behavior by one person may facilitate the occurrence of subsequent, similar behaviors by others. The process is implemented via imitation. Theories of imitation have been postulated to explain clustering of suicides and DSH behaviors. Studies conducted primarily in adolescents revealed that up to 5 percent of all suicides may be the result of suicide clustering and that exposure to DSH behaviors in family and friends was predictive of DSH and suicide ideation. A large body of research in the last 10 years clearly demonstrated that extensive newspaper and television coverage of suicide is associated with a significant increase in the rate of suicide. The magnitude of the increase is proportional to the amount, duration, and prominence of the media coverage. This phenomenon is termed the "Werther effect" after Goethe's novel, *The Sorrows of Young Werther* (1774), which was assumed to have triggered an increase in suicides after its release. As a result, the book was banned in many European countries. Today, the increasing popularity of the Internet as a source of information has raised concerns about the danger of sites that promote suicide and sites set up by strangers who form suicide pacts. Further empirical research is needed to clarify their effects. By the same token, however, the media may also serve as an effective means for preventing suicide contagion. More efforts should be directed at presenting stories of suicide, especially by persons admired by youth, in a different light. One successful example is the media's treatment of the suicide of the guitarist and singer, Kurt Cobain. The lack of an apparent copycat effect following Cobain's death is hypothesized to be due to various aspects of the media coverage and the intense activity of the crisis center and community outreach interventions in Seattle that occurred following Cobain's suicide.

Preventive Measures

Despite the heavy burden that adolescent suicidal behavior imposes on individuals and communities, little is known about effective preventive measures. Of the few studies that have investigated such interventions, most were targeted at adults and reported only moderate effectiveness. More attention is now being addressed at school-based prevention programs, which hold particular promise because teachers and other school staff can serve as "gatekeepers" or "gateway providers," spotting students who seem to be in turmoil and referring them to mental health services. This approach is noteworthy because the latest research suggests that most suicidal youth do not receive mental healthcare or even tell an adult about their suicidal thoughts or behaviors. Furthermore, there are many innovative prevention efforts directed at ethnic minorities in which suicidal behavior has become epidemic, such as native Indians of Arizona and the Inuit in Canada. They focus on restoring ethnic pride and cultural values using a "bottom-up" approach, starting with intensive consultation with the local community. Further research is needed to understand the phenomenology of suicidal behaviors among ethnic minority populations, including the presentations of suicidal behavior, meanings of suicidal behavior in different cultures, risk factors particular to these groups and their correlates, applicability of known risk factors in other populations, such as depression, and preventive mechanisms.

Chapter 7
Firearms And Suicide

Nearly two-thirds of the 32,000 gun deaths in the United States are suicides, according to the latest data from the Centers for Disease Control and Prevention (CDC). Firearm suicides outnumber firearm homicides nearly two to one. Indeed, far more Americans die by turning a gun on themselves than at the hands of others.

> Firearms are the leading method of suicide, accounting for half of all suicide deaths. The reason is that guns are more lethal than other suicide methods. About 85 percent of suicide attempts with a gun are fatal, whereas only 2 percent of overdoses, the most widely used method in suicide attempts, end in death. Clearly, suicide method is a crucial factor in determining whether a suicide attempt will be fatal.

Suicide attempts are often impulsive and triggered by an immediate crisis, such as the loss of a job or the breakup of a relationship. While most suicidal impulses are intense, they typically last only a short period of time. Intervention during this time of acute risk is critical. The vast majority—90 percent—of people who attempt suicide and survive do not go on to die by suicide. Suicide attempts with a gun, however, rarely afford a second chance. In addition to being highly lethal, firearms leave little opportunity for rescue or to halt mid-attempt. Limiting access to firearms increases the amount of time between a crisis and an individual's suicide attempt, giving the impulse an opportunity to pass.

Research shows there is a clear connection between firearms in the home and an increased risk of suicide. People who live in a home with a gun are three times more likely to die by

About This Chapter: This chapter includes text excerpted from "The Truth About Suicide & Guns," © 2017 The Brady Center to Prevent Gun Violence. Reprinted with permission. For the full article please visit www.bradycampaign.org/sites/default/files/Brady-Guns-Suicide-Report-2016.pdf

suicide than those without access. Within the United States, suicide rates, both overall and by firearm, are higher in places where household firearm ownership is more common.

Firearm Suicide In The United States

Suicide is the 10th leading cause of death in the United States and second among adolescents and young adults aged 10 to 24 years. Each year, more than 39,000 people die by suicide in the United States, half (51 percent) by using a firearm.

The risk of firearm suicide varies greatly by age, sex, and race. Rates increase significantly with age and are highest among adults age 70 and older; 74 percent of suicides among this age group involve firearms. However, nearly two-thirds (62 percent) of firearm suicide deaths are among people ages 55 and younger. Notably, although adolescents and young adults ages 10 to 24 years do not have the highest rates of suicide, the impact is high relative to other causes of death. More young people die each year from suicide than from cancer, heart disease, AIDS, birth defects, strokes, pneumonia and influenza, and chronic lung diseases combined. The majority of young people who die by suicide use a firearm (44 percent).

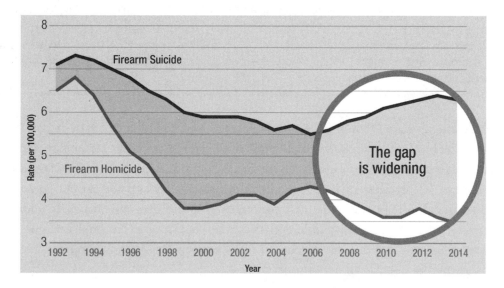

Figure 7.1. Trends in Firearm-Related Death Rates 1992–2014*

* 2014 is the most recent year for which data are available. Data were obtained from the CDC Web-based Injury Statistics Query and Reporting System, which lags two years behind the current year.

Regardless of age or race, men have the highest rates of firearm suicide. Men account for 87 percent of all firearm suicide deaths and have a rate nearly seven times higher than that of women (11.21 and 1.61 per 100,000, respectively).

Overall, whites have the highest rates of firearm suicide, followed by American Indians and Alaska Natives (7.03 and 4.37 per 100,000, respectively). However, some important exceptions exist. Among 15- to 19-year-olds and 20- to 24-year-olds, American Indians and Alaska Natives have the highest rates of firearm suicide. Even so, whites account for 93 percent of all firearm suicide deaths.

The Link Between Suicide And Guns

There is overwhelming evidence linking firearm availability and suicide risk. More than a dozen U.S. case control studies, performed over the last 25 years, have examined this relationship. All of them reached the same conclusion: firearms in the home are associated with significantly higher rates of suicide.

Studies examining firearm ownership and suicide rates at the national, state, and regional levels provide further evidence of the firearm-suicide connection. They show that suicide rates, both overall and by firearm, are higher in areas where gun ownership is more widespread. One study investigated the association between firearm prevalence and suicide at the state level using firearm ownership data from the Behavioral Risk Factor Surveillance System. The study found that states with the highest firearm prevalence had 1.9 times more suicide deaths and 3.8 times more firearm suicide deaths than states with the lowest firearm prevalence. This relationship persisted even after taking into account other factors that could influence suicide rates, such as mental illness, alcohol dependence or abuse, illicit substance dependence or abuse, unemployment, and poverty rates.

Three factors are at the root of the effect guns have on suicide deaths. First, the wide availability of firearms in the United States increases the likelihood that a suicide attempt will occur. Second is the high lethality of firearms, which means a suicidal person has less opportunity for survival and is less likely to be interrupted while attempting suicide. Finally, because most suicides are highly impulsive, the quick, easy, and destructive nature of firearm injury means those who decide to attempt suicide with a firearm in the midst of a crisis are less able to fully consider their decision and change their mind.

Availability

A number of factors can influence an individual's choice of suicide method. However, the ready availability of and the individual's familiarity with a suicide method have been shown to be particularly important factors in the decision. In the United States, where guns are widely available, firearms are the most common suicide method.

> Firearm ownership is more prevalent in the United States than in any other country; the number of privately owned firearms is estimated to be between 270 million and 310 million.

By many measures, about one-third of American households own a firearm, with gun ownership just as common in households with children as those without. Twenty-two percent of adults report personally owning a gun; the vast majority are white, male, and over the age of 50.

Surveys have found that storage practices vary among gun owners. A national study showed that fewer than half (39 percent) of households with children store their guns unloaded and locked, with ammunition stored separately. A separate study estimated that nearly two million children live in homes that have unlocked and loaded firearms.

Lethality

Compared with the other most commonly used suicide methods, firearm suicides are the most fatal. Firearms make death a much more likely result for a suicide attempt: 85 to 91 percent of firearm suicide attempts are fatal compared with 3 percent or less for some of the other most commonly used methods, such as overdosing and wrist cutting. As presented in Figure 7.2, firearms are used in more than half of all suicides.

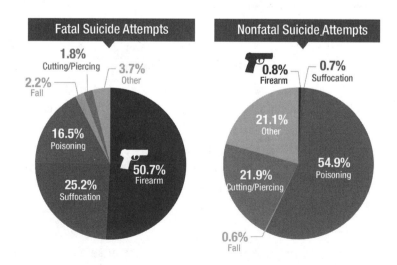

Figure 7.2. Fatal and Nonfatal Suicide Attempts by Method (5 year)

Suicide attempts involving guns are over 45 times more fatal than attempts involving overdosing, around 30 times more fatal than those involving cutting or stabbing, and almost three times more fatal than suicide attempts by jumping. Moreover, unlike other methods, suicide with a firearm is easy and requires little planning. Individuals attempting suicide by this method do not have an opportunity to reconsider or halt mid-attempt.

Women attempt suicide up to three times more often than men but have significantly lower rates of suicide death. Men are four times more likely than women to die by suicide. As Figure 7.3 shows, this result is obtained because guns are the suicide method of choice for men. In comparison, women are more likely to choose less lethal methods, such as pills.

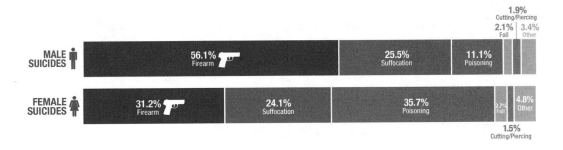

Figure 7.3. Suicide Deaths by Method (5 year)

Impulsivity

Although some suicide attempts are carefully planned, many are impulsive. Various studies of survivors of suicide have calculated that as many as two-thirds of those who reported suicidal behavior did not plan their attempt. Interviews with survivors of near-lethal suicide attempts revealed that a quarter made the attempt less than five minutes after making the decision. About half of those did so within 20 minutes, and three-quarters of suicide attempts occurred within an hour. In a separate study, survivor interviews found that many made their attempt within 24 hours of a crisis, particularly interpersonal crises and physical fights.

Limiting Access To Lethal Means

The research presented thus far convincingly demonstrates that ready availability of a firearm increases the likelihood of suicide. Given this stark connection, making firearms less available would seem to be a logical strategy for prevention. Since many suicides are impulsive, separating someone from the means to self-harm takes away their ability to act on what otherwise might have been a fleeting impulse. Suicidal crises are often triggered by an immediate stressor, such as the loss of a job or the breakup of a relationship. However, the urge to act is fairly short-lived, typically lasting a few minutes to a few hours. That's why delaying access to a gun is critical; it allows time for the suicidal impulse to pass without being realized.

Intervention during this time of acute risk is key to saving lives. Most people who attempt suicide don't really want to die, they are just so overwhelmed by their emotions they feel unable to cope. Indeed, the vast majority of people who make it through a suicidal crisis do not go on to die by suicide. A systematic review of 70 studies following patients after a non-fatal attempt found that, on average, only 7 percent (range: 5 to 11 percent) eventually died by suicide, whereas 70 percent did not attempt again. A common misconception is that people who want to die will find a way to kill themselves, with or without a gun. However, studies suggest that the risk of method substitution is low. If a person's preferred suicide method is unavailable, it is unlikely they will switch to a different one. Even if another method is used it is likely to be less lethal, thus increasing the odds of survival.

Opportunities For Prevention

According to the World Health Organization's global report on suicide prevention, "Restriction of access to means plays an important role in suicide prevention, particularly in the case of suicides that are impulsive." In the 2012 *National Strategy for Suicide Prevention*, a joint report issued by the U.S. Surgeon General and the National Action Alliance for Suicide Prevention, one of the 11 goals outlined was to "promote efforts to reduce access to lethal means of suicide among individuals with identified suicide risk."

Parents Of Adolescents And Young Adults

Suicide is the second leading cause of death for adolescents and young adults 10 to 24 years of age in the United States. Firearms, used in 44 percent of cases, are the most common method of suicide for this age group.

Studies show that young people often have easy access to the guns they use to kill themselves. In fact, compared to households with younger children, households with adolescents are more likely to store a firearm loaded and unlocked. Most parents of adolescents believe their children are old enough to behave responsibly and to exercise good judgment around guns.

However, the vast majority (82 percent) of firearm suicides among adolescents involve a gun belonging to a family member; roughly 75 percent use a parent's gun.

A review of data from case-control studies reveals that adolescents who died by suicide were four to five times more likely to have a gun in the home, even after adjusting for potentially confounding variables, such as previous mental health problems. Although suicide and mental illness can be closely related, 40 percent of suicide completers under the age of 16 were found to have no known psychiatric disorder. For young people without mental illness, a loaded gun in the home was found to increase suicide risk 32 times. These data show that for many young people the availability of a gun in the home is the most significant predictor of suicide.

Educating parents about lethal means reduction should be an important part of any effort to prevent adolescent suicide. Many parents are unaware of the risks of having a gun in the home, particularly for older adolescents. Therefore, parents should be encouraged to store household firearms safely (locked and unloaded, with ammunition stored separately) or to remove them altogether. In one study, keeping guns locked and unloaded was found to have a protective effect, reducing odds of death by 73 percent and 70 percent, respectively. However, removing firearms from the home is the most reliable and most effective way to prevent youth suicide.

Healthcare Providers

Healthcare providers are in a unique position to reach people in crisis, particularly those at risk for suicide. Nearly half (45 percent) of people who died by suicide had contact with a primary care provider in the month before their death, and 77 percent had contact within a year. Many people in crisis also seek care in hospital emergency departments. In fact, suicide attempts represent a growing proportion of emergency department visits. In addition, a large number of patients who visit emergency rooms for reasons unrelated to mental health also suffer depression and have suicidal thoughts. However, emergency departments are often underused in suicide prevention.

The fact that few emergency room providers counsel patients on lethal means reduction is undoubtedly related to the misconceptions many have about suicide. A survey of emergency room providers found that less than half believed suicide was preventable. Although over half of providers agreed that emergency room staff have a responsibility to counsel patients on reducing access to lethal means, only 81 percent of physicians and 67 percent of nurses reported they would counsel a patient on lethal means in cases where the patient had a suicide plan involving a firearm. Visits with healthcare providers represent critical opportunities to intervene before a suicide attempt. The 2012 *National Strategy for Suicide Prevention* recommends that providers routinely ask about the presence of lethal means (including firearms and medications) in the home and educate about ways to minimize associated risks. Studies have shown that parents of at-risk youth seen in an emergency department were more likely to lock up firearms if they received counseling from a healthcare provider.

Firearms Dealers And Firing Range Owners

Research has shown that the time immediately following a firearm purchase is a particularly high-risk period for suicide. A study of handgun sales in California found that suicide was the leading cause of death for handgun purchasers in the year following purchase. In the first week after purchase, the firearm suicide rate among purchasers was 57 times higher than that of the general population. This statistic plainly shows that some firearms are bought for the purpose of carrying out a suicide.

By intervening in sales where customers show signs of distress or crisis, firearms dealers and firing range owners can play a crucial role in preventing suicide. Recent purchases of handguns account for 10 percent of all suicides by firearm. However, this figure does not take into account the full impact of a handgun purchase, which has been shown to nearly double the suicide risk for other members of the household. Gun shops are in a unique position to educate gun owners on the risks of keeping guns in the home and the steps they can take to mitigate them.

Chapter 8
Attitudes About Mental Health

Stigma And Mental Illness

Stigma has been defined as an attribute that is deeply discrediting. This stigmatized trait sets the bearer apart from the rest of society, bringing with it feelings of shame and isolation. Often, when a person with a stigmatized trait is unable to perform an action because of the condition, other people view the person as the problem rather than viewing the condition as the problem. More recent definitions of stigma focus on the results of stigma—the prejudice, avoidance, rejection and discrimination directed at people believed to have an illness, disorder or other trait perceived to be undesirable. Stigma causes needless suffering, potentially causing a person to deny symptoms, delay treatment and refrain from daily activities. Stigma can exclude people from access to housing, employment, insurance, and appropriate medical care. Thus, stigma can interfere with prevention efforts, and examining and combating stigma is a public health priority.

The Substance Abuse and Mental Health Services Administration (SAMHSA) and the Centers for Disease Control and Prevention (CDC) have examined public attitudes toward mental illness in two surveys. In the 2006 HealthStyles survey, only one-quarter of young adults between the ages of 18–24 believed that a person with mental illness can eventually recover. In 2007, adults in 37 states and territories were surveyed about their attitudes toward

About This Chapter: Text under the heading "Stigma And Mental Illness" is excerpted from "Mental Health Basics," Centers for Disease Control and Prevention (CDC), June 18, 2015; Text under the heading "Mental Health Myths And Facts" is excerpted from "Mental Health Myths And Facts," MentalHealth.gov, U.S. Department of Health and Human Services (HHS) May 31, 2013. Reviewed January 2017; Text under the heading "Attitudes And Discrimination" is excerpted from "Attitudes And Discrimination," Youth.gov, November 1, 2012. Reviewed January 2017.

mental illness, using the 2007 Behavioral Risk Factor Surveillance System (BRFSS) Mental Illness and Stigma module. This study found that:

- 78 percent of adults with mental health symptoms and 89 percent of adults without such symptoms agreed that treatment can help persons with mental illness lead normal lives.

- 57 percent of adults without mental health symptoms believed that people are caring and sympathetic to persons with mental illness.

- Only 25 percent of adults with mental health symptoms believed that people are caring and sympathetic to persons with mental illness.

These findings highlight both the need to educate the public about how to support persons with mental illness and the need to reduce barriers for those seeking or receiving treatment for mental illness.

Mental Health Myths And Facts

Can you tell the difference between a mental health myth and fact?

Mental Health Problems Affect Everyone

Myth: Mental health problems don't affect me.

Fact: Mental health problems are actually very common. In 2014, about:

- One in five American adults experienced a mental health issue

- One in 10 young people experienced a period of major depression

- One in 25 Americans lived with a serious mental illness, such as schizophrenia, bipolar disorder, or major depression

Suicide is the 10th leading cause of death in the United States. It accounts for the loss of more than 41,000 American lives each year, more than double the number of lives lost to homicide.

Myth: Children don't experience mental health problems.

Fact: Even very young children may show early warning signs of mental health concerns. These mental health problems are often clinically diagnosable, and can be a product of the interaction of biological, psychological, and social factors.

Half of all mental health disorders show first signs before a person turns 14 years old, and three quarters of mental health disorders begin before age 24.

Unfortunately, less than 20 percent of children and adolescents with diagnosable mental health problems receive the treatment they need. Early mental health support can help a child before problems interfere with other developmental needs.

Myth: People with mental health problems are violent and unpredictable.

Fact: The vast majority of people with mental health problems are no more likely to be violent than anyone else. Most people with mental illness are not violent and only 3–5 percent of violent acts can be attributed to individuals living with a serious mental illness. In fact, people with severe mental illnesses are over 10 times more likely to be victims of violent crime than the general population. You probably know someone with a mental health problem and don't even realize it, because many people with mental health problems are highly active and productive members of our communities.

Myth: People with mental health needs, even those who are managing their mental illness, cannot tolerate the stress of holding down a job.

Fact: People with mental health problems are just as productive as other employees. Employers who hire people with mental health problems report good attendance and punctuality as well as motivation, good work, and job tenure on par with or greater than other employees.

When employees with mental health problems receive effective treatment, it can result in:

- lower total medical costs
- increased productivity
- lower absenteeism
- decreased disability costs

Myth: Personality weakness or character flaws cause mental health problems. People with mental health problems can snap out of it if they try hard enough.

Fact: Mental health problems have nothing to do with being lazy or weak and many people need help to get better. Many factors contribute to mental health problems, including:

- Biological factors, such as genes, physical illness, injury, or brain chemistry
- Life experiences, such as trauma or a history of abuse
- Family history of mental health problems

People with mental health problems can get better and many recover completely.

Helping Individuals with Mental Health Problems

Myth: There is no hope for people with mental health problems. Once a friend or family member develops mental health problems, he or she will never recover.

Fact: Studies show that people with mental health problems get better and many recover completely. Recovery refers to the process in which people are able to live, work, learn, and participate fully in their communities. There are more treatments, services, and community support systems than ever before, and they work.

Myth: Therapy and self-help are a waste of time. Why bother when you can just take a pill?

Fact: Treatment for mental health problems varies depending on the individual and could include medication, therapy, or both. Many individuals work with a support system during the healing and recovery process.

Myth: I can't do anything for a person with a mental health problem.

Fact: Friends and loved ones can make a big difference. Only 44 percent of adults with diagnosable mental health problems and less than 20 percent of children and adolescents receive needed treatment. Friends and family can be important influences to help someone get the treatment and services they need by:

- reaching out and letting them know you are available to help
- helping them access mental health services
- learning and sharing the facts about mental health, especially if you hear something that isn't true
- treating them with respect, just as you would anyone else
- refusing to define them by their diagnosis or using labels such as "crazy"

Myth: Prevention doesn't work. It is impossible to prevent mental illnesses.

Fact: Prevention of mental, emotional, and behavioral disorders focuses on addressing known risk factors such as exposure to trauma that can affect the chances that children, youth, and young adults will develop mental health problems. Promoting the social-emotional well-being of children and youth leads to:

- higher overall productivity
- better educational outcomes
- lower crime rates

- stronger economies

- lower healthcare costs

- improved quality of life

- increased lifespan

- improved family life

Attitudes And Discrimination

Discrimination against youth with mental health challenges begins early and increases over time, causing attitudes to become ingrained. Despite the fact that an overwhelming majority of Americans believe that people with mental illnesses are not to blame for their conditions (84%), only about 57.3 percent believe that people are generally caring and sympathetic toward individuals with mental illnesses. This percentage is much lower (24.6%) for those who themselves suffer poor mental health.

Attitudes Of Young People

Discrimination and misconceptions about people with mental illnesses is prevalent for youth and young adults. Findings from the 2006 HealthStyles Survey suggest that, for young adults between the ages of 18 and 24,

- about 24 percent believe that a person with a mental illness is dangerous and 38.9 percent believe he or she is unpredictable;

- less than half (44.3%) believe that someone with a mental illness can be successful at work;

- only slightly more than half (55.2%) believe that treatment can help people with mental illnesses lead normal lives; and

- only around 26.9 percent believe that a person with mental illness can eventually recover.

Discrimination As A Barrier To Recovery

Discrimination associated with mental illness poses a large barrier to recovery and is one of the main reasons why people don't seek help and treatment. Further, an unwillingness to seek help because of the negative attitudes attached to mental health and substance abuse disorders or to suicidal thoughts has been found to be one of the risk factors associated with suicide.

What Can Be Done To Limit Discrimination?

Youth are a key population on which to focus discrimination reduction efforts, as they are more likely than the general public to know someone with a mental illness, and therefore have a unique opportunity to make a difference. The National Annenberg Survey of Youth conducted a large scale study on these negative attitudes and found that youth who were informed with facts and able to dispel myths about individuals with mental health disorders were less likely to discriminate against them. They concluded that various approaches have promise in decreasing negative attitudes and discrimination, such as the use of mass media to influence the attitudes of youth and educating students by incorporating persons with mental health disorders as speakers in classroom presentations and discussions.

SAMHSA suggests everyone can do something to help a person with mental illness by

- avoiding the use of negative labels;

- showing kindness and respect; and

- helping to eliminate discrimination in housing, employment, or education.

In addition, understanding and accepting friends play an important role in recovery.

- Friends can help by offering reassurance, companionship, and emotional strength.

- Friends can express an interest and concern for people with a mental illness by asking questions, listening to ideas, and being responsive.

- Friends can help encourage others to treat mental illness like any other healthcare condition.

- Friends can dismiss any preconceived notions about mental illness and embrace a more helpful way of relating to people.

Chapter 9
Suicide Among LGBT Youth

Behavioral Health Of Lesbian, Gay, Bisexual And Transgender (LGBT) Youth

"Behavioral health" is an umbrella term that includes issues and services related to both mental health and substance use. Information relevant to these two areas have been synthesized below.

Mental Health And Suicide

As the Institute of Medicine has noted, LGBT youth are typically well adjusted and mentally healthy. However, they experience higher rates of mental health challenges and increased health complications arising from these challenges compared to their heterosexual peers. Research on transgender youth outcomes as separate from lesbian, gay, and bisexual youth outcomes is more limited, though growing. Some recent nonrandom surveys of self-identified transgender people indicate that up to one-third reported attempting suicide at least once, with higher rates for youth and young adults than for older adults. Moreover, suicide is the third leading cause of death among youth ages 15 to 24, and LGBT youth are more likely to attempt suicide than their peers. This does not mean, however, that LGBT identity itself is the cause of these challenges. Rather, these higher rates may be due to bias, discrimination, family rejection, and other stressors associated with how they are treated because of their sexual identity or gender identity/expression. These challenges, which researchers refer to as

About This Chapter: Text under the heading "Behavioral Health Of Lesbian, Gay, Bisexual And Transgender Youth" is excerpted from "Behavioral Health," Youth.gov, July 1, 2014; Text under the heading "Lesbian, Gay, And Bisexual High School Students' Health" is excerpted from "First National Study Of Lesbian, Gay, And Bisexual High School Students' Health," Centers for Disease Control and Prevention (CDC), August 11, 2016.

"microaggresions," can contribute to anxiety, depression, and other mental health challenges, as well as to suicide and self-harming behavior.

Research has found that lesbian, gay, and bisexual youth have much higher levels of suicidal ideation than their heterosexual peers. Also, recent population-based studies suggest that the reported rates of suicide attempts for high school students who identify as LGBT are two to seven times higher than rates among high school students who describe themselves as heterosexual. LGBT youth are also twice as likely to have thoughts about suicide. The 2009 Youth Risk Behavior Surveillance System found that during the 12 months before the survey was administered, across the sites evaluated,

- the percentage of students who reported having felt sad or hopeless ranged from 19.3 percent to 29.0 percent among heterosexual students, from 28.8 percent to 52.8 percent among lesbian and gay students, and from 47.2 percent to 62.9 percent among bisexual students;

- the percentage of students who seriously considered attempting suicide ranged from 9.9 percent to 13.2 percent for heterosexual students, but from 18.8 percent to 43.4 percent among lesbian and gay students; and

- the percentage of students who attempted suicide one or more times ranged from 3.8 percent to 9.6 percent among heterosexual students, but from 15.1 percent to 34.3 percent among lesbian and gay students.

Strategies to improve mental health and prevent self-harming behavior and suicide include

- providing safe and supportive environments, particularly through affirming relationships with family and peers;

- enacting legislation to protect the safety of LGBT youth;

- re-evaluating institutional practices that undermine positive child and youth development; and

- building community awareness and capacity to understand and address stressors that LGBT youth may experience.

Substance Use

LGBT youth may be more likely to use substances to cope with bias and stress and may be more likely to experience increased rates of depression and anxiety than their non-LGBT peers. Challenges such as family rejection of, or anticipated reaction to, one's LGBT identity are also associated with substance use. For example, one study found that youth who experienced a moderate level of family rejection were 1.5 times more likely to use illegal substances than those who experienced little to no rejection; youth experiencing high levels of family rejection were 3.5 times more likely to use these substances. Also, youth who have run away from home have higher rates of alcohol and illicit drug use.

Additionally, an analysis of more than 18 studies between 1994 and 2006 examining the use of tobacco, alcohol, and illicit drugs (e.g., methamphetamines, marijuana) found that lesbian, gay, and bisexual youth had higher rates of usage for all these substances than their heterosexual peers. Lesbian and bisexual girls were 9.7 times more likely than heterosexual girls to smoke cigarettes, and a quarter of young gay men reported regular binge drinking.

Transgender youth have a high risk for developing substance dependency issues. Transgender people have higher rates of usage for some drugs and may have higher rates of methamphetamine, injectable drug, and tobacco usage. Additionally, transgender youth face more barriers to accessing behavioral healthcare. These barriers include experiencing physical/verbal abuse by other clients and staff; being required to wear clothing based on their sex rather than their identified gender; and being required to shower/sleep in areas based on their sex rather than their identified gender. Providers with culturally and linguistically competent practices can help improve the quality of care for transgender youth and address these barriers.

Reducing the rates of bias, discrimination, and victimization that LGBT youth experience can help reduce substance use. A related strategy includes creating safe spaces for LGBT youth in drug-free environments such as community centers. Also, accepting/positive family behaviors toward LGBT youth during adolescence can protect against not only suicide and depression but also substance use.

Lesbian, Gay, And Bisexual High School Students' Health

The first nationally representative study of U.S. lesbian, gay, and bisexual high school students finds that lesbian, gay, and bisexual students experience substantially higher levels of physical and sexual violence and bullying than other students.

Accelerated Action Needed To Protect Vulnerable Youth

The report, Sexual Identity, Sex of Sexual Contacts, and Health-Related Behaviors Among Students in Grades 9–12—United States and Selected Sites, 2015, found that compared to their heterosexual peers, these students are significantly more likely to report:

- Being physically forced to have sexual intercourse (18 percent lesbian/gay/bisexual vs. 5 percent heterosexual)

- Experiencing sexual dating violence (23 percent lesbian/gay/bisexual vs. 9 percent heterosexual)

- Experiencing physical dating violence (18 percent lesbian/gay/bisexual vs. 8 percent heterosexual)

- Being bullied at school or online (at school: 34 percent lesbian/gay/bisexual vs. 19 percent heterosexual; online: 28 percent lesbian/gay/bisexual vs. 14 percent heterosexual)

"Quantifying these risks and negative outcomes on a national scale is critical to protect the health and well-being of more than one million lesbian, gay, and bisexual high school students," said Jonathan Mermin, M.D., director of CDC's National Center for HIV/AIDS, Viral Hepatitis, STD, and TB Prevention. "These tragic disparities call for accelerated action by public health and education agencies, communities, and families to protect the lives of lesbian, gay and bisexual youth."

The report, in CDC's Morbidity and Mortality Weekly Report (MMWR), compares the prevalence of more than 100 health behaviors among lesbian, gay, and bisexual students to the prevalence of these behaviors among heterosexual students. These analyses are possible due to the inclusion of two new questions about sex of sexual contacts and sexual identity on the 2015 National Youth Risk Behavior Survey (YRBS). The YRBS is the nation's principal source of data for tracking national health risk behaviors among high school students.

"These findings confirm substantial disparities in violence-related and other health risk behaviors among students who identify as lesbian, gay, and bisexual," said Laura Kann, Ph.D., chief of the School-Based Surveillance Branch within CDC's Division of Adolescent and School Health. "While smaller studies have shown similar disparities, this study documents the national scope of the problem and will open the door to the type of analyses, research, and programs needed to protect the next generation."

Lesbian, Gay, And Bisexual Youth At High Risk For Suicide And Other Severe Outcomes

While physical and sexual violence and bullying are serious health dangers on their own, a combination of complex factors can place young people at high risk for suicide, depression, addiction, poor academic performance, and other severe consequences.

The YRBS data show lesbian, gay and bisexual students are at substantial risk for several of these serious outcomes:

- More than 40 percent of lesbian, gay, and bisexual students have seriously considered suicide, and 29 percent reported having attempted suicide during the past 12 months.

- Sixty percent of lesbian, gay, and bisexual students reported having been so sad or hopeless they stopped doing some of their usual activities.

- Lesbian, gay, and bisexual students are up to five times more likely than other students to report using illegal drugs.

- More than one in 10 lesbian, gay, and bisexual students reported missing school during the past 30 days due to safety concerns. While not a direct measure of school performance, absenteeism has been linked to low graduation rates, which can have lifelong consequences.

"Unfortunately, the YRBS data don't tell us why we see these disparities, but other research points to issues that may put youth at risk for sexual and physical abuse and other types of violence," said Deb Houry, M.D., M.P.H., director of CDC's National Center for Injury Prevention and Control. "These include social isolation, lack of parental or caregiver support, or not being perceived as being masculine or feminine enough."

Parents, Schools, And Communities Can Serve As Sources Of Strength

Research suggests that comprehensive, community-wide prevention efforts can reduce the risk of multiple types of violence for these and other vulnerable youth. Studies suggest that parents can play a role in fostering resiliency by providing strong family support and teaching all adolescents non-violent problem-solving skills. Schools can also build an environment that provides a sense of safety and connection for all students, including lesbian, gay, and bisexual youth.

"Connectedness—or social bonds—to peers, teachers, schools, or community organizations is key to protecting the health of these adolescents," said Mermin. "Students will succeed if they know they matter, and feel safe and supported socially, emotionally, and physically. Solutions may not be simple, but we can take action to build support for lesbian, gay and bisexual youth at multiple levels."

CDC works with communities, schools, and partners across the nation to expand programs and support data collection and research on the most effective approaches to prevent sexual, dating, and other types of violence and provide the support needed to protect victims from suicide and other severe consequences. Among key efforts, CDC is working to expand available data on suicide, to provide resources and support to schools in violence and bullying prevention, and to evaluate numerous community-level programs to prevent youth violence.

"Tragically, when young people face multiple types of violence or other adverse events in childhood, especially in the absence of support from family, peers, and communities, the consequences can be life-threatening," said Houry. "All of us can help to position lesbian, gay, and bisexual youth to survive and thrive in their environments, and it's critical that we take action."

The Youth Risk Behavior Surveillance System is one of several key CDC surveillance systems collecting health-related data on lesbian, gay, and bisexual individuals. Another critical effort is the expansion of the National Violent Death Reporting System, which provides rich information about the circumstances of violent deaths. In 2012, CDC added available data on sexual orientation and gender identity to the system. While the system is not yet available in every state, CDC is currently collecting these data from 32 states. These data help fill an important gap in information on death from suicide—information public health officials believe is critical to understand and ultimately address factors that lead to suicide.

To reach and protect youth in school settings, CDC provides tools, expertise, and support to education partners across the nation as they work to promote healthy environments, including prohibiting violence and bullying, ensuring students have access to caring adults, and improving health and education services to meet the needs of lesbian, gay, bisexual, and other vulnerable youth.

CDC is also working to evaluate several approaches to suicide and other violence prevention in youth. Programs being implemented and evaluated focus on a number of factors, including school-based social and emotional learning, individual problem solving skills, and community mentorship and other support systems.

Part Two
Mental Health Disorders And Life-Threatening Behaviors Linked To Suicide Risk

Chapter 10
Depression: A Key Risk For Suicide

Feeling moody, sad, or grouchy? Who doesn't once in a while? But if you have been feeling sad, hopeless, or irritable for at least 2 weeks, you might have depression. You're not alone. You should know:

- Depression is a medical illness.

- Depression can be treated.

- Early treatment is best.

What Is Depression?

Depression is a medical illness with many symptoms, including physical ones. Sadness is only a small part of depression. Some people with depression may not feel sadness at all, but be more irritable, or just lose interest in things they usually like to do. Depression interferes with your daily life and normal function. Don't ignore or try to hide the symptoms. It is not a character flaw, and you can't will it away.

Are There Different Types Of Depression?

Yes. The most common depressive disorders include major depression (a discrete episode, clearly different from a person's usual feeling and functioning), persistent depressive disorder (a chronic, low-grade depression that can get better or worse over time), and psychotic depression (the most severe, with delusions or hallucinations). Some people are

About This Chapter: This chapter includes text excerpted from "Depression And College Students," National Institute of Mental Health (NIMH), November 2015.

vulnerable to depression in the winter ("seasonal affective disorder"), and some women report depression in the week or two prior to their menstrual period ("premenstrual dysphoric disorder").

What Are The Signs And Symptoms Of Depression?

If you have been experiencing any of the following signs and symptoms nearly every day for at least 2 weeks, you may have major (sometimes called "clinical") depression:

- Persistent sad, anxious, or "empty" mood

- Feelings of hopelessness, pessimism

- Feelings of guilt, worthlessness, helplessness

- Loss of interest or pleasure in hobbies and activities

- Decreased energy, fatigue, being "slowed down"

- Difficulty concentrating, remembering, making decisions

- Difficulty sleeping, early-morning awakening, or oversleeping

- Appetite and/or unwanted weight changes

- Thoughts of death or suicide; suicide attempts

- Restlessness, irritability

- Persistent physical symptoms, such as muscle pain or headaches

Not everyone who is depressed experiences every symptom. Some people experience only a few symptoms. Some people have many. *If any of these symptoms is interfering with your functioning—or if you are having thoughts that life is not worth living or ideas of harming yourself—you should seek help immediately; it is not necessary to wait 2 weeks.*

What Are "Co-Occurring" Disorders?

Depression can occur at the same time as other health problems, such as anxiety, an eating disorder, or substance abuse. It can also co-occur with other medical conditions, such as diabetes or thyroid imbalance. Certain medications—for example, those for the treatment of severe acne—may cause side effects that contribute to depression; although some women are very sensitive to hormonal changes, modern birth control pills are not associated with depression for most users.

If I Think I May Have Depression, Where Can I Get Help?

If you have symptoms of depression that are getting in the way of your ability to function with your studies and your social life, ask for help. Depression can get better with care and treatment. Don't wait for depression to go away by itself or think you can manage it all on your own, and don't ignore how you're feeling just because you think you can "explain" it. As a college student, you're busy—but you need to make time to get help. If you don't ask for help, depression may get worse and contribute to other health problems, while robbing you of the academic and social enjoyment and success that brought you to college in the first place. It can also lead to "self-medication" with high-risk behaviors with their own serious consequences, such as binge drinking and other substance abuse and having unsafe sex.

Most colleges provide mental health services through counseling centers, student health centers, or both. Check out your college website for information. If you think you might have depression, start by making an appointment with a doctor or healthcare provider for a checkup. This can be a doctor or healthcare provider at your college's student health services center, a doctor who is off-campus in your college town, or a doctor in your hometown. Your doctor can make sure that you do not have another health problem that is causing your depression.

If your doctor finds that you do not have another health problem, he or she can discuss treatment options or refer you to a mental health professional, such as a psychiatrist, counselor, or psychologist. A mental health professional can give you a thorough evaluation and also treat your depression.

If you have thoughts of wishing you were dead or of suicide, call a helpline, such as 800-273-TALK (800-273-8255), for free 24-hour help, call campus security or 911, or go to the nearest emergency room.

Depression, A Major Risk Factor For Suicide

Depression is also a major risk factor for suicide. The following are some of the signs you might notice in yourself or a friend that may be reason for concern.

- Talking about wanting to die or to kill oneself
- Looking for a way to kill oneself, such as searching online or buying a gun
- Talking about feeling hopeless or having no reason to live

- Talking about feeling trapped or in unbearable pain
- Talking about being a burden to others and that others would be better off if one was gone
- Increasing the use of alcohol or drugs
- Acting anxious or agitated; behaving recklessly
- Giving away prized possessions
- Sleeping too little or too much
- Withdrawing or feeling isolated
- Showing rage or talking about seeking revenge
- Displaying extreme mood swings

What Should I Do If I Am Considering Suicide?

If you are in crisis and need help, call this toll-free number, available 24 hours a day, every day: 800-273-TALK (800-273-8255). You will reach the National Suicide Prevention Lifeline, a service available to anyone. You may call for yourself or for someone you care about, and all calls are confidential. You can also visit the Lifeline's website at www.suicidepreventionlifeline.org.

What Should I Do If Someone I Know Is Considering Suicide?

If you know someone who is considering suicide, do not leave him or her alone. Try to get your friend or loved one to seek immediate help from his or her doctor, campus security, the student health service, or the nearest hospital emergency room, or call 911. Remove any access he or she may have to firearms or other potential tools for suicide, including medications. You can also call to seek help as soon as possible by calling the Lifeline at 800-273-TALK (800-273-8255).

Chapter 11

How Is Depression Detected And Treated?

Depression Is Treatable

If you think you may have depression, start by making an appointment to see your doctor or healthcare provider. This could be your primary doctor or a health provider who specializes in diagnosing and treating mental health conditions (psychologist or psychiatrist). Certain medications, and some medical conditions, such as viruses or a thyroid disorder, can cause the same symptoms as depression. A doctor can rule out these possibilities by doing a physical exam, interview, and lab tests. If the doctor can find no medical condition that may be causing the depression, the next step is a psychological evaluation.

Talking To Your Doctor

How well you and your doctor talk to each other is one of the most important parts of getting good healthcare. But talking to your doctor isn't always easy. It takes time and effort on your part as well as your doctor's.

To prepare for your appointment, make a list of:

- **Any symptoms you've had,** including any that may seem unrelated to the reason for your appointment

- When did your symptoms start?

About This Chapter: Text under the heading "Depression Is Treatable" is excerpted from "Depression: What You Need To Know," National Institute of Mental Health (NIMH), 2015; Text under the heading "Treatment And Therapies" is excerpted from "Depression," National Institute of Mental Health (NIMH), October 2016. Text under the heading "What Else Can I Do?" is excerpted from "Depression And College Students," National Institute of Mental Health (NIMH), November 2015.

- How severe are your symptoms?

- Have the symptoms occurred before?

- If the symptoms have occurred before, how were they treated?

- **Key personal information,** including any major stresses or recent life changes

- **All medications, vitamins,** or other supplements that you're taking, including how much and how often

- **Questions to ask** your health provider

If you don't have a primary doctor or are not at ease with the one you currently see, now may be the time to find a new doctor. Whether you just moved to a new city, changed insurance providers, or had a bad experience with your doctor or medical staff, it is worthwhile to spend time finding a doctor you can trust.

Tests And Diagnosis

Your doctor or healthcare provider will examine you and talk to you at the appointment. Your doctor may do a physical exam and ask questions about your health and symptoms. There are no lab tests that can specifically diagnose depression, but your doctor may also order some lab tests to rule out other conditions.

Ask questions if the doctor's explanations or instructions are unclear, bring up problems even if the doctor doesn't ask, and let the doctor know if you have concerns about a particular treatment or change in your daily life.

Your doctor may refer you to a mental health professional, such as a psychiatrist, psychologist, social worker, or mental health counselor, who should discuss with you any family history of depression or other mental disorder, and get a complete history of your symptoms. The mental health professional may also ask if you are using alcohol or drugs, and if you are thinking about death or suicide.

Treatment And Therapies

Depression, even the most severe cases, can be treated. The earlier that treatment can begin, the more effective it is. Depression is usually treated with medications, psychotherapy, or a combination of the two. If these treatments do not reduce symptoms, electroconvulsive therapy (ECT) and other brain stimulation therapies may be options to explore.

> **Quick Tip**
>
> No two people are affected the same way by depression and there is no "one-size-fits-all" for treatment. It may take some trial and error to find the treatment that works best for you.

Medications

Antidepressants are medicines that treat depression. They may help improve the way your brain uses certain chemicals that control mood or stress. You may need to try several different antidepressant medicines before finding the one that improves your symptoms and has manageable side effects. A medication that has helped you or a close family member in the past will often be considered.

Antidepressants take time—usually 2 to 4 weeks—to work, and often, symptoms such as sleep, appetite, and concentration problems improve before mood lifts, so it is important to give medication a chance before reaching a conclusion about its effectiveness. If you begin taking antidepressants, do not stop taking them without the help of a doctor. Sometimes people taking antidepressants feel better and then stop taking the medication on their own, and the depression returns. When you and your doctor have decided it is time to stop the medication, usually after a course of 6 to 12 months, the doctor will help you slowly and safely decrease your dose. Stopping them abruptly can cause withdrawal symptoms.

> **Remember!!**
>
> In some cases, children, teenagers, and young adults under 25 may experience an increase in suicidal thoughts or behavior when taking antidepressants, especially in the first few weeks after starting or when the dose is changed. This warning from the U.S. Food and Drug Administration (FDA) also says that patients of all ages taking antidepressants should be watched closely, especially during the first few weeks of treatment.
>
> If you are considering taking an antidepressant and you are pregnant, planning to become pregnant, or breastfeeding, talk to your doctor about any increased health risks to you or your unborn or nursing child.
>
> To find the latest information about antidepressants, talk to your doctor and visit www.fda.gov.

You may have heard about an herbal medicine called St. John's wort. Although it is a top-selling botanical product, the FDA has not approved its use as an over-the-counter or prescription medicine for depression, and there are serious concerns about its safety (it should never be combined with a prescription antidepressant) and effectiveness. Do not use St. John's wort before talking to your healthcare provider. Other natural products sold as dietary supplements, including omega-3 fatty acids and S-adenosylmethionine (SAMe), remain under study but have not yet been proven safe and effective for routine use.

Psychotherapies

Several types of psychotherapy (also called "talk therapy" or, in a less specific form, counseling) can help people with depression. Examples of evidence-based approaches specific to the treatment of depression include cognitive-behavioral therapy (CBT), interpersonal therapy (IPT), and problem-solving therapy.

Brain Stimulation Therapies

If medications do not reduce the symptoms of depression, electroconvulsive therapy (ECT) may be an option to explore. Based on the latest research:

- ECT can provide relief for people with severe depression who have not been able to feel better with other treatments.

- Electroconvulsive therapy can be an effective treatment for depression. In some severe cases where a rapid response is necessary or medications cannot be used safely, ECT can even be a first-line intervention.

- Once strictly an inpatient procedure, today ECT is often performed on an outpatient basis. The treatment consists of a series of sessions, typically three times a week, for two to four weeks.

- ECT may cause some side effects, including confusion, disorientation, and memory loss. Usually these side effects are short-term, but sometimes memory problems can linger, especially for the months around the time of the treatment course. Advances in ECT devices and methods have made modern ECT safe and effective for the vast majority of patients. Talk to your doctor and make sure you understand the potential benefits and risks of the treatment before giving your informed consent to undergoing ECT.

- ECT is not painful, and you cannot feel the electrical impulses. Before ECT begins, a patient is put under brief anesthesia and given a muscle relaxant. Within one hour after the treatment session, which takes only a few minutes, the patient is awake and alert.

Other more recently introduced types of brain stimulation therapies used to treat medicine-resistant depression include repetitive transcranial magnetic stimulation (rTMS) and vagus nerve stimulation (VNS). Other types of brain stimulation treatments are under study.

Beyond Treatment: Things You Can Do

Here are other tips that may help you or a loved one during treatment for depression:

- Try to be active and exercise.

- Set realistic goals for yourself.

- Try to spend time with other people and confide in a trusted friend or relative.

- Try not to isolate yourself, and let others help you.

- Expect your mood to improve gradually, not immediately.

- Postpone important decisions, such as getting married or divorced, or changing jobs until you feel better. Discuss decisions with others who know you well and have a more objective view of your situation.

- Continue to educate yourself about depression.

What Else Can I Do?

Besides seeing a doctor and a counselor, you can also help your depression by being patient with yourself and good to yourself. Don't expect to get better immediately, but you will feel yourself improving gradually over time.

- Daily exercise, spending time outside in nature and in the sun, and eating healthy foods can also help you feel better.

- Get enough sleep. Try to have consistent sleep habits and avoid all-night study sessions.

- Your counselor may teach you how to be aware of your feelings and teach you relaxation techniques. Use these when you start feeling down or upset.

- Avoid using drugs and at least minimize, if not totally avoid, alcohol.

- Break up large tasks into small ones, and do what you can as you can; try not to do too many things at once.

- Try to spend time with supportive family members or friends, and take advantage of campus resources, such as student support groups. Talking with your parents, guardian, or other students who listen and care about you gives you support.

- Try to get out with friends and try fun things that help you express yourself. As you recover from depression, you may find that even if you don't feel like going out with friends, if you push yourself to do so, you'll be able to enjoy yourself more than you thought.

Remember that, by treating your depression, you are helping yourself succeed in college and after graduation.

Chapter 12
Dealing With Teen Depression

What Is Depression?

If you have been feeling sad, hopeless, or irritable for what seems like a long time, you might have depression.

- Depression is a real, treatable brain illness, or health problem.

- Depression can be caused by big transitions in life, stress, or changes in your body's chemicals that affect your thoughts and moods.

- Even if you feel hopeless, depression gets better with treatment.

- There are lots of people who understand and want to help you.

- Ask for help as early as you can so you can get back to being yourself.

Regular Sadness And Depression Are Not The Same

Regular Sadness

Feeling moody, sad, or grouchy? Who doesn't once in a while? It's easy to have a couple of bad days. Your schoolwork, activities, and family and friend drama, all mixed with not enough sleep, can leave you feeling overwhelmed. On top of that, teen hormones can be all over the place and also make you moody or cry about the smallest thing. Regular moodiness and sadness usually go away quickly though, within a couple of days.

About This Chapter: This chapter includes text excerpted from "Teen Depression," National Institute of Mental Health (NIMH), 2015.

Depression

Untreated depression is a more intense feeling of sadness, hopelessness, and anger or frustration that lasts much longer, such as for weeks, months, or longer. These feelings make it hard for you to function as you normally would or participate in your usual activities. You may also have trouble focusing and feel like you have little to no motivation or energy. You may not even feel like seeing your best friends. Depression can make you feel like it is hard to enjoy life or even get through the day.

If You Think You Are Depressed, Ask For Help As Early As You Can

If you have symptoms of depression for more than 2 weeks, ask for help. Depression can get better with care and treatment. Don't wait for depression to go away by itself. If you don't ask for help, depression may get worse.

1. **Talk to:**

   - your parents or guardian

   - your teacher or counselor

   - your doctor

   - a helpline, such as 800-273-TALK (800-273-8255), free 24-hour help

   - or call 911 if you are in a crisis or want to hurt yourself.

2. **Ask your parent or guardian to make an appointment with your doctor for a checkup.** Your doctor can make sure that you do not have another health problem that is causing your depression. If your doctor finds that you do not have another health problem, he or she can treat your depression or refer you to a mental health professional. A mental health professional can give you a thorough evaluation and also treat your depression.

3. **Talk to a mental health professional, such as a psychiatrist, counselor, psychologist, or other therapist.** These mental health professionals can diagnose and treat depression and other mental health problems.

Know The Signs And Symptoms Of Depression

Most of the day or nearly every day you may feel one or all of the following:

- Sad

- Empty

- Hopeless

- Angry, cranky, or frustrated, even at minor things

You also may:

- Not care about things or activities you used to enjoy.

- Have weight loss when you are not dieting or weight gain from eating too much.

- Have trouble falling asleep or staying asleep, or sleep much more than usual.

- Move or talk more slowly.

- Feel restless or have trouble sitting still.

- Feel very tired or like you have no energy.

- Feel worthless or very guilty.

- Have trouble concentrating, remembering information, or making decisions.

- Think about dying or suicide or try suicide.

Not everyone experiences depression the same way. And depression can occur at the same time as other mental health problems, such as anxiety, an eating disorder, or substance abuse.

There Are Ways You Can Feel Better

Effective treatments for depression include talk therapy or a combination of talk therapy and medicine.

Talk Therapy

A therapist, such as a psychiatrist, a psychologist, a social worker, or counselor can help you understand and manage your moods and feelings. You can talk out your emotions to someone who understands and supports you. You can also learn how to stop thinking negatively and start to look at the positives in life. This will help you build confidence and feel better about yourself. Research has shown that certain types of talk therapy or psychotherapy can help teens deal with depression. These include cognitive behavioral therapy, which focuses on thoughts, behaviors, and feelings related to depression, and interpersonal psychotherapy, which focuses on working on relationships.

Medicines

If your doctor thinks you need medicine to help your depression, he or she can prescribe an antidepressant. There are a few antidepressants that have been widely studied and proven to help teens. If your doctor recommends medicine, it is important to see your doctor regularly and tell your parents or guardian about your feelings, especially if you start feeling worse or have thoughts of hurting yourself.

Using Antidepressants

Here are some things to remember about using antidepressants:

- **Get a prescription.**

   Antidepressants are prescription medications. Talk to your healthcare provider if you want to take antidepressants. If your doctor writes you a prescription for an antidepressant, ask exactly how you should take the medication. There are many types of antidepressants, so you and your doctor have options to choose from. Sometimes, it takes trying several different medications to find the best one for you. If you are worried about cost, ask your doctor or pharmacist if the medication comes in a generic form. Generic medications can cost less than brand names.

- **Be patient.**

   When taking these antidepressants, it is important to stick with them for a while. Many people start feeling better a few days after starting the medication. But it often takes several weeks of taking an antidepressant to feel a big difference. Maybe a month or more to feel the most benefit. It's also common to have to change the dose, so you will want to work closely with your doctor.

- **Talk about timing.**

   How long someone takes antidepressants differs from person to person. Many people take them for 6–12 months, and some people take them for a longer time. Talk to your doctor about a timeline that works for you.

- **Ask about side effects.**

   Antidepressants are safe and work well for most people. But it is still important to talk with your doctor about side effects you may get. Side effects usually do not get in the way of daily life, and they may go away as your body gets used to the medication.

If you notice that your mood is getting worse, especially if you have thoughts about hurting yourself, it is important to call your doctor right away.

(Source: "Using Antidepressants," Smokefree Women, U.S. Department of Health and Human Services (HHS).)

Be Good To Yourself

Besides seeing a doctor and a counselor, you can also help your depression by being patient with yourself and good to yourself. Don't expect to get better immediately, but you will feel yourself improving gradually over time.

- Daily exercise, getting enough sleep, spending time outside in nature and in the sun, or eating healthy foods can also help you feel better.

- Your counselor may teach you how to be aware of your feelings and teach you relaxation techniques. Use these when you start feeling down or upset.

- Try to spend time with supportive family members. Talking with your parents, guardian, or other family members who listen and care about you gives you support and they can make you laugh.

- Try to get out with friends and try fun things that help you express yourself.

Depression Can Affect Relationships

It's understandable that you don't want to tell other people that you have been struggling with depression. But know that depression can affect your relationships with family and friends, and how you perform at school. Maybe your grades have dropped because you find it hard to concentrate and stay on top of school. Teachers may think that you aren't trying in class. Maybe because you're feeling hopeless, peers think you are too negative and start giving you a hard time.

Know that their misunderstanding won't last forever because you are getting better with treatment. Think about talking with people you trust to help them understand what you are going through.

Depression Is Not Your Fault Or Caused By Something You Did Wrong

Depression is a real, treatable brain illness, or health problem. Depression can be caused by big transitions in life, stress, or changes in your body's chemicals that affect your thoughts and moods. Depression can run in families. Maybe you haven't realized that you have depression and have been blaming yourself for being negative. Remember that depression is not your fault!

Chapter 13
Bipolar Disorder

What Is Bipolar Disorder?

Bipolar disorder is a serious brain illness. It is also called manic-depressive illness or manic depression. Children with bipolar disorder go through unusual mood changes. Sometimes they feel very happy or "up," and are much more energetic and active than usual, or than other kids their age. This is called a **manic episode.** Sometimes children with bipolar disorder feel very sad and "down," and are much less active than usual. This is called depression or a **depressive episode.**

Bipolar disorder is not the same as the normal ups and downs every kid goes through. Bipolar symptoms are more powerful than that. The mood swings are more extreme and are accompanied by changes in sleep, energy level, and the ability to think clearly. Bipolar symptoms are so strong, they can make it hard for a child to do well in school or get along with friends and family members. The illness can also be dangerous. Some young people with bipolar disorder try to hurt themselves or attempt suicide.

Children and teens with bipolar disorder should get treatment. With help, they can manage their symptoms and lead successful lives.

Who Develops Bipolar Disorder?

Anyone can develop bipolar disorder, including children and teens. However, most people with bipolar disorder develop it in their late teen or early adult years. The illness usually lasts a lifetime.

About This Chapter: This chapter includes text excerpted from "Bipolar Disorder In Children And Teens," National Institute of Mental Health (NIMH), 2015.

Why Does Someone Develop Bipolar Disorder?

Doctors do not know what causes bipolar disorder, but several things may contribute to the illness. Family genes may be one factor because bipolar disorder sometimes runs in families. However, it is important to know that just because someone in your family has bipolar disorder, it does not mean other members of the family will have it as well.

Another factor that may lead to bipolar disorder is the brain structure or the brain function of the person with the disorder. Scientists are finding out more about the disorder by studying it. This research may help doctors do a better job of treating people. Also, this research may help doctors to predict whether a person will get bipolar disorder. One day, doctors may be able to prevent the illness in some people.

What Are The Symptoms Of Bipolar Disorder?

Bipolar "mood episodes" include unusual mood changes along with unusual sleep habits, activity levels, thoughts, or behavior. In a child, these mood and activity changes must be very different from their usual behavior and from the behavior of other children. A person with bipolar disorder may have manic episodes, depressive episodes, or "mixed" episodes. A mixed episode has both manic and depressive symptoms. These mood episodes cause symptoms that last a week or two or sometimes longer. During an episode, the symptoms last every day for most of the day.

Children and teens having a manic episode may:

- feel very happy or act silly in a way that's unusual for them and for other people their age

- have a very short temper

- talk really fast about a lot of different things

- have trouble sleeping but not feel tired

- have trouble staying focused

- talk and think about sex more often

- do risky things

Children and teens having a depressive episode may:

- feel very sad

- complain about pain a lot, such as stomachaches and headaches

- sleep too little or too much

- feel guilty and worthless

- eat too little or too much

- have little energy and no interest in fun activities

- think about death or suicide

Can Children And Teens With Bipolar Disorder Have Other Problems?

Young people with bipolar disorder can have several problems at the same time. These include:

- **Substance abuse.** Both adults and kids with bipolar disorder are at risk of drinking or taking drugs.

- **Attention deficit hyperactivity disorder (ADHD).** Children who have both bipolar disorder and ADHD may have trouble staying focused.

- **Anxiety disorders,** like separation anxiety.

Sometimes behavior problems go along with mood episodes. Young people may take a lot of risks, such as driving too fast or spending too much money. Some young people with bipolar disorder think about suicide. **Watch for any signs of suicidal thinking. Take these signs seriously and call your child's doctor.**

Bipolar Disorder And Co-Occurring Substance Use Disorders

Research suggests that from 30 percent to more than 50 percent of people with bipolar disorder will develop a substance use disorder (SUD) sometime during their lives. This co-occurrence complicates the course, diagnosis, and treatment of SUDs. However, treatment for bipolar disorder and SUDs is available, and remission and recovery are possible—especially with early intervention.

Alcohol is commonly misused by people with bipolar disorder, and people with bipolar disorder and co-occurring alcohol use disorder are less likely to respond and adhere to treatment and more likely to be hospitalized and to attempt suicide than people with bipolar disorder only. In some cases, the combination of bipolar disorder and an SUD may deepen bipolar disorder's manic and depressive symptoms.

(Source: "An Introduction To Bipolar Disorder And Co-Occurring Substance Use Disorders," Substance Abuse and Mental Health Services Administration (SAMHSA).)

How Is Bipolar Disorder Diagnosed?

An experienced doctor will carefully examine your child. There are no blood tests or brain scans that can diagnose bipolar disorder. Instead, the doctor will ask questions about your child's mood and sleeping patterns. The doctor will also ask about your child's energy and behavior. Sometimes doctors need to know about medical problems in your family, such as depression or alcoholism. The doctor may use tests to see if something other than bipolar disorder is causing your child's symptoms.

How Is Bipolar Disorder Treated?

Right now, there is no cure for bipolar disorder. Doctors often treat children who have the illness in much the same way they treat adults. Treatment can help control symptoms. Steady, dependable treatment works better than treatment that starts and stops. Treatment options include:

- **Medication.** There are several types of medication that can help. Children respond to medications in different ways, so the right type of medication depends on the child. Some children may need more than one type of medication because their symptoms are so complex. Sometimes they need to try different types of medicine to see which are best for them. Children should take the fewest number of medications and the smallest doses possible to help their symptoms. A good way to remember this is "start low, go slow."

- **Therapy.** Different kinds of psychotherapy, or "talk" therapy, can help children with bipolar disorder. Therapy can help children change their behavior and manage their routines. It can also help young people get along better with family and friends. Sometimes therapy includes family members.

> Medications can cause side effects. **Always tell your child's doctor about any problems with side effects.** Do not stop giving your child medication without a doctor's help. Stopping medication suddenly can be dangerous, and it can make bipolar symptoms worse.

What Can Children And Teens Expect From Treatment?

With treatment, children and teens with bipolar disorder can get better over time. It helps when doctors, parents, and young people work together.

Sometimes a child's bipolar disorder changes. When this happens, treatment needs to change too. For example, your child may need to try a different medication. The doctor may also recommend other treatment changes. Symptoms may come back after a while, and more adjustments may be needed. Treatment can take time, but sticking with it helps many children and teens have fewer bipolar symptoms.

You can help treatment be more effective. Try keeping a chart of your child's moods, behaviors, and sleep patterns. This is called a "daily life chart" or "mood chart." It can help you and your child understand and track the illness. A chart can also help the doctor see whether treatment is working.

Personal Story

James has bipolar disorder.

Here's his story.

Four months ago, James found out he has bipolar disorder. He knows it's a serious illness, but he was relieved when he found out. That's because he had symptoms for years, but no one knew what was wrong. Now he's getting treatment and feeling better.

James often felt really sad. As a kid, he skipped school or stayed in bed when he was down. At other times, he felt really happy. He talked fast and felt like he could do anything. James lived like this for a long time, but things changed last year. His job got very stressful. He felt like he was having more "up" and "down" times. His wife and friends wanted to know what was wrong. He told them to leave him alone and said everything was fine.

A few weeks later, James couldn't get out of bed. He felt awful, and the bad feelings went on for days. Then, his wife took him to the family doctor, who sent James to a psychiatrist. He talked to this doctor about how he was feeling. Soon James could see that his ups and downs were serious. He was diagnosed with bipolar disorder, and he started treatment.

These days, James takes medicine and goes to talk therapy. Treatment was hard at first, and recovery took some time, but now he's back at work. His mood changes are easier to handle, and he's having fun again with his wife and friends.

(Source: "Bipolar Disorder," National Institute of Mental Health (NIMH).)

How Does Bipolar Disorder Affect Parents And Family?

Taking care of a child or teenager with bipolar disorder can be stressful for you, too. You have to cope with the mood swings and other problems, such as short tempers and risky activities. This can challenge any parent. Sometimes the stress can strain your relationships with other people, and you may miss work or lose free time.

If you are taking care of a child with bipolar disorder, take care of yourself too. Find someone you can talk to about your feelings. Talk with the doctor about support groups for caregivers. If you keep your stress level down, you will do a better job. It might help your child get better too.

How Can I Help My Child Or Teen?

Help begins with the right diagnosis and treatment. If you think your child may have bipolar disorder, make an appointment with your family doctor to talk about the symptoms you notice.

If your child has bipolar disorder, here are some basic things you can do:

- Be patient.

- Encourage your child to talk, and listen to your child carefully.

- Be understanding about mood episodes.

- Help your child have fun.

- Help your child understand that treatment can make life better.

Where Do I Go For Help?

If you're not sure where to get help, call your family doctor. You can also check the phone book for mental health professionals. Hospital doctors can help in an emergency. Finally, the Substance Abuse and Mental Health Services Administration (SAMHSA) has an online tool to help you find mental health services in your area. You can find it here: findtreatment.samhsa.gov.

Chapter 14
Anxiety Disorders

Occasional anxiety is a normal part of life. You might feel anxious when faced with a problem at work, before taking a test, or making an important decision. But anxiety disorders involve more than temporary worry or fear. For a person with an anxiety disorder, the anxiety does not go away and can get worse over time. The feelings can interfere with daily activities such as job performance, school work, and relationships. There are several different types of anxiety disorders. Examples include generalized anxiety disorder, panic disorder, and social anxiety disorder.

Childhood anxiety disorders are very common, affecting one in eight children. The National Institute of Mental Health (NIMH) estimates a lifetime prevalence between the ages 13 and 18 years of 25.1 percent and a lifetime prevalence of 5.9 percent for "severe" anxiety disorder. Anxiety disorders in childhood generally follow an unremitting course leading to additional psychopathology and often interfere with social, emotional, and academic development. Early intervention is especially important given the childhood onset and unrelenting course of anxiety disorders.

(Source: "Anxiety in Children," Agency for Healthcare Research and Quality (AHRQ), U.S. Department of Health and Human Services (HHS).)

Signs And Symptoms
Generalized Anxiety Disorder

People with generalized anxiety disorder display excessive anxiety or worry for months and face several anxiety-related symptoms.

About This Chapter: This chapter includes text excerpted from "Anxiety Disorders," National Institute of Mental Health (NIMH), March 2016.

Generalized anxiety disorder symptoms include:

- Restlessness or feeling wound-up or on edge

- Being easily fatigued

- Difficulty concentrating or having their minds go blank

- Irritability

- Muscle tension

- Difficulty controlling the worry

- Sleep problems (difficulty falling or staying asleep or restless, unsatisfying sleep)

Panic Disorder

People with panic disorder have recurrent unexpected panic attacks, which are sudden periods of intense fear that may include palpitations, pounding heart, or accelerated heart rate; sweating; trembling or shaking; sensations of shortness of breath, smothering, or choking; and feeling of impending doom.

Panic disorder symptoms include:

- Sudden and repeated attacks of intense fear

- Feelings of being out of control during a panic attack

- Intense worries about when the next attack will happen

- Fear or avoidance of places where panic attacks have occurred in the past

Social Anxiety Disorder

People with social anxiety disorder (sometimes called "social phobia") have a marked fear of social or performance situations in which they expect to feel embarrassed, judged, rejected, or fearful of offending others.

Social anxiety disorder symptoms include:

- Feeling highly anxious about being with other people and having a hard time talking to them

- Feeling very self-conscious in front of other people and worried about feeling humiliated, embarrassed, or rejected, or fearful of offending others

- Being very afraid that other people will judge them

- Worrying for days or weeks before an event where other people will be

- Staying away from places where there are other people

- Having a hard time making friends and keeping friends

- Blushing, sweating, or trembling around other people

- Feeling nauseous or sick to your stomach when other people are around

Evaluation for an anxiety disorder often begins with a visit to a primary care provider. Some physical health conditions, such as an overactive thyroid or low blood sugar, as well as taking certain medications, can imitate or worsen an anxiety disorder. A thorough mental health evaluation is also helpful, because anxiety disorders often co-exist with other related conditions, such as depression or obsessive-compulsive disorder.

Risk Factors

Researchers are finding that genetic and environmental factors, frequently in interaction with one another, are risk factors for anxiety disorders. Specific factors include:

- shyness, or behavioral inhibition, in childhood

- being female

- having few economic resources

- being divorced or widowed

- exposure to stressful life events in childhood and adulthood

- anxiety disorders in close biological relatives

- parental history of mental disorders

- elevated afternoon cortisol levels in the saliva (specifically for social anxiety disorder)

Bullying, Anxiety, And Suicide

Negative outcomes of bullying (for youth who bully others, youth who are bullied, and youth who both are bullied and bully others) may include: depression, anxiety, involvement in interpersonal violence or sexual violence, substance abuse, poor social functioning, and poor school performance, including lower grade point averages, standardized test scores, and poor attendance.

> Youth who report both being bullied and bullying others (sometimes referred to as bully-victims) have the highest rates of negative mental health outcomes, including depression, anxiety, and thinking about suicide.
>
> *(Source: "The Relationship Between Bullying And Suicide: What We Know And What It Means For Schools," Centers for Disease Control and Prevention (CDC).)*

Treatments And Therapies

Anxiety disorders are generally treated with psychotherapy, medication, or both.

Psychotherapy

Psychotherapy or "talk therapy" can help people with anxiety disorders. To be effective, psychotherapy must be directed at the person's specific anxieties and tailored to his or her needs. A typical "side effect" of psychotherapy is temporary discomfort involved with thinking about confronting feared situations.

Cognitive Behavioral Therapy (CBT)

CBT is a type of psychotherapy that can help people with anxiety disorders. It teaches a person different ways of thinking, behaving, and reacting to anxiety-producing and fearful situations. CBT can also help people learn and practice social skills, which is vital for treating social anxiety disorder.

Two specific stand-alone components of CBT used to treat social anxiety disorder are **cognitive therapy** and **exposure therapy.** Cognitive therapy focuses on identifying, challenging, and then neutralizing unhelpful thoughts underlying anxiety disorders.

Exposure therapy focuses on confronting the fears underlying an anxiety disorder in order to help people engage in activities they have been avoiding. Exposure therapy is used along with relaxation exercises and/or imagery. One study, called a meta-analysis because it pulls together all of the previous studies and calculates the statistical magnitude of the combined effects, found that cognitive therapy was superior to exposure therapy for treating social anxiety disorder.

CBT may be conducted individually or with a group of people who have similar problems. Group therapy is particularly effective for social anxiety disorder. Often "homework" is assigned for participants to complete between sessions.

Self-Help Or Support Groups

Some people with anxiety disorders might benefit from joining a self-help or support group and sharing their problems and achievements with others. Internet chat rooms might also be useful, but any advice received over the Internet should be used with caution, as Internet acquaintances have usually never seen each other and false identities are common. Talking with a trusted friend or member of the clergy can also provide support, but it is not necessarily a sufficient alternative to care from an expert clinician.

Stress Management Techniques

Stress management techniques and meditation can help people with anxiety disorders calm themselves and may enhance the effects of therapy. While there is evidence that aerobic exercise has a calming effect, the quality of the studies is not strong enough to support its use as treatment. Since caffeine, certain illicit drugs, and even some over-the-counter cold medications can aggravate the symptoms of anxiety disorders, avoiding them should be considered. Check with your physician or pharmacist before taking any additional medications.

The family can be important in the recovery of a person with an anxiety disorder. Ideally, the family should be supportive but not help perpetuate their loved one's symptoms.

Medication

Medication docs not cure anxiety disorders but often relieves symptoms. Medication can only be prescribed by a medical doctor (such as a psychiatrist or a primary care provider), but a few states allow psychologists to prescribe psychiatric medications.

Medications are sometimes used as the initial treatment of an anxiety disorder, or are used only if there is insufficient response to a course of psychotherapy. In research studies, it is common for patients treated with a combination of psychotherapy and medication to have better outcomes than those treated with only one or the other.

The most common classes of medications used to combat anxiety disorders are antidepressants, anti-anxiety drugs, and beta blockers. Be aware that some medications are effective only if they are taken regularly and that symptoms may recur if the medication is stopped.

Antidepressants

Antidepressants are used to treat depression, but they also are helpful for treating anxiety disorders. They take several weeks to start working and may cause side effects such as headache, nausea, or difficulty sleeping. The side effects are usually not a problem for most people, especially if the dose starts off low and is increased slowly over time.

> **Please Note:** Although antidepressants are safe and effective for many people, they may be risky for children, teens, and young adults. A "black box" warning—the most serious type of warning that a prescription can carry—has been added to the labels of antidepressants. The labels now warn that antidepressants may cause some people to have suicidal thoughts or make suicide attempts. For this reason, anyone taking an antidepressant should be monitored closely, especially when they first start taking the medication.

Anti-Anxiety Medications

Anti-anxiety medications help reduce the symptoms of anxiety, panic attacks, or extreme fear and worry. The most common anti-anxiety medications are called benzodiazepines. Benzodiazepines are first-line treatments for generalized anxiety disorder. With panic disorder or social phobia (social anxiety disorder), benzodiazepines are usually second-line treatments, behind antidepressants.

Beta Blockers

Beta blockers, such as propranolol and atenolol, are also helpful in the treatment of the physical symptoms of anxiety, especially social anxiety. Physicians prescribe them to control rapid heartbeat, shaking, trembling, and blushing in anxious situations.

Choosing the right medication, medication dose, and treatment plan should be based on a person's needs and medical situation, and done under an expert's care. Only an expert clinician can help you decide whether the medication's ability to help is worth the risk of a side effect. Your doctor may try several medicines before finding the right one.

You and your doctor should discuss:

- How well medications are working or might work to improve your symptoms

- Benefits and side effects of each medication

- Risk for serious side effects based on your medical history

- The likelihood of the medications requiring lifestyle changes

- Costs of each medication

- Other alternative therapies, medications, vitamins, and supplements you are taking and how these may affect your treatment

- How the medication should be stopped. Some drugs can't be stopped abruptly but must be tapered off slowly under a doctor's supervision

Chapter 15
Schizophrenia And Suicide

What Is Schizophrenia?

Schizophrenia is a chronic and severe disorder that affects how a person thinks, feels, and acts. Although schizophrenia is not as common as other mental disorders, it can be very disabling. Approximately 7 or 8 individuals out of 1,000 will have schizophrenia in their lifetime.

People with the disorder may hear voices or see things that aren't there. They may believe other people are reading their minds, controlling their thoughts, or plotting to harm them. This can be scary and upsetting to people with the illness and make them withdrawn or extremely agitated. It can also be scary and upsetting to the people around them.

People with schizophrenia may sometimes talk about strange or unusual ideas, which can make it difficult to carry on a conversation. They may sit for hours without moving or talking. Sometimes people with schizophrenia seem perfectly fine until they talk about what they are really thinking.

Families and society are impacted by schizophrenia too. Many people with schizophrenia have difficulty holding a job or caring for themselves, so they may rely on others for help. Stigmatizing attitudes and beliefs about schizophrenia are common and sometimes interfere with people's willingness to talk about and get treatment for the disorder.

People with schizophrenia may cope with symptoms throughout their lives, but treatment helps many to recover and pursue their life goals. Researchers are developing more effective treatments and using new research tools to understand the causes of schizophrenia. In the years to come, this work may help prevent and better treat the illness.

About This Chapter: This chapter includes text excerpted from "Schizophrenia," National Institute of Mental Health (NIMH), 2015.

What Are The Symptoms Of Schizophrenia?

The symptoms of schizophrenia fall into three broad categories: positive, negative, and cognitive symptoms.

Positive Symptoms

Positive symptoms are psychotic behaviors not generally seen in healthy people. People with positive symptoms may "lose touch" with some aspects of reality. For some people, these symptoms come and go. For others, they stay stable over time. Sometimes they are severe, and at other times hardly noticeable. The severity of positive symptoms may depend on whether the individual is receiving treatment. Positive symptoms include the following:

Hallucinations are sensory experiences that occur in the absence of a stimulus. These can occur in any of the five senses (vision, hearing, smell, taste, or touch). "Voices" (auditory hallucinations) are the most common type of hallucination in schizophrenia. Many people with the disorder hear voices. The voices can either be internal, seeming to come from within one's own mind, or they can be external, in which case they can seem to be as real as another person speaking. The voices may talk to the person about his or her behavior, command the person to do things, or warn the person of danger. Sometimes the voices talk to each other, and sometimes people with schizophrenia talk to the voices that they hear. People with schizophrenia may hear voices for a long time before family and friends notice the problem.

Other types of hallucinations include seeing people or objects that are not there, smelling odors that no one else detects, and feeling things like invisible fingers touching their bodies when no one is near.

Delusions are strongly held false beliefs that are not consistent with the person's culture. Delusions persist even when there is evidence that the beliefs are not true or logical. People with schizophrenia can have delusions that seem bizarre, such as believing that neighbors can control their behavior with magnetic waves. They may also believe that people on television are directing special messages to them, or that radio stations are broadcasting their thoughts aloud to others. These are called "delusions of reference."

Sometimes they believe they are someone else, such as a famous historical figure. They may have paranoid delusions and believe that others are trying to harm them, such as by cheating, harassing, poisoning, spying on, or plotting against them or the people they care about. These beliefs are called "persecutory delusions."

Thought disorders are unusual or dysfunctional ways of thinking. One form is called "disorganized thinking." This is when a person has trouble organizing his or her thoughts or connecting them logically. He or she may talk in a garbled way that is hard to understand. This is often called "word salad." Another form is called "thought blocking." This is when a person stops speaking abruptly in the middle of a thought. When asked why he or she stopped talking, the person may say that it felt as if the thought had been taken out of his or her head. Finally, a person with a thought disorder might make up meaningless words, or "neologisms."

Movement disorders may appear as agitated body movements. A person with a movement disorder may repeat certain motions over and over. In the other extreme, a person may become catatonic. Catatonia is a state in which a person does not move and does not respond to others. Catatonia is rare today, but it was more common when treatment for schizophrenia was not available.

Negative Symptoms

Negative symptoms are associated with disruptions to normal emotions and behaviors. These symptoms are harder to recognize as part of the disorder and can be mistaken for depression or other conditions. These symptoms include the following:

- "Flat affect" (reduced expression of emotions via facial expression or voice tone)
- Reduced feelings of pleasure in everyday life
- Difficulty beginning and sustaining activities
- Reduced speaking

People with negative symptoms may need help with everyday tasks. They may neglect basic personal hygiene.

This may make them seem lazy or unwilling to help themselves, but the problems are symptoms caused by schizophrenia.

Cognitive Symptoms

For some people, the cognitive symptoms of schizophrenia are subtle, but for others, they are more severe and patients may notice changes in their memory or other aspects of thinking. Similar to negative symptoms, cognitive symptoms may be difficult to recognize as part of the disorder. Often, they are detected only when specific tests are performed. Cognitive symptoms include the following:

- Poor "executive functioning" (the ability to understand information and use it to make decisions)

- Trouble focusing or paying attention
- Problems with "working memory" (the ability to use information immediately after learning it)

Poor cognition is related to worse employment and social outcomes and can be distressing to individuals with schizophrenia.

When Does Schizophrenia Start, And Who Gets It?

Schizophrenia affects slightly more males than females. It occurs in all ethnic groups around the world. Symptoms such as hallucinations and delusions usually start between ages 16 and 30. Males tend to experience symptoms a little earlier than females. Most commonly, schizophrenia occurs in late adolescence and early adulthood. It is uncommon to be diagnosed with schizophrenia after age 45. Schizophrenia rarely occurs in children, but awareness of childhood-onset schizophrenia is increasing.

It can be difficult to diagnose schizophrenia in teens. This is because the first signs can include a change of friends, a drop in grades, sleep problems, and irritability—behaviors that are common among teens. A combination of factors can predict schizophrenia in up to 80 percent of youth who are at high risk of developing the illness. These factors include isolating oneself and withdrawing from others, an increase in unusual thoughts and suspicions, and a family history of psychosis. This pre-psychotic stage of the disorder is called the "prodromal" period.

Prevalence Of Schizophrenia

Worldwide prevalence estimates range between 0.5 percent and 1.0 percent. Age of first episode is typically younger among men (about 21 years of age) than women (27 years). Of persons with schizophrenia, by age 30, 9 out of 10 men, but only 2 out of 10 women, will manifest the illness.

(Source: "Mental Health: Burden of Mental Illness," Centers for Disease Control and Prevention (CDC).)

Are People With Schizophrenia Violent?

Most people with schizophrenia are not violent. In fact, most violent crimes are not committed by people with schizophrenia. People with schizophrenia are much more likely to harm themselves than others. Substance abuse may increase the chance a person will become violent. The risk of violence is greatest when psychosis is untreated and decreases substantially when treatment is in place.

Schizophrenia And Suicidal Thoughts

Suicidal thoughts and behaviors are very common among people with schizophrenia. People with schizophrenia die earlier than people without a mental illness, partly because of the increased suicide risk.

It is hard to predict which people with schizophrenia are more likely to die by suicide, but actively treating any co-existing depressive symptoms and substance abuse may reduce suicide risk. People who take their antipsychotic medications as prescribed are less likely to attempt suicide than those who do not. If someone you know is talking about or has attempted suicide, help him or her find professional help right away or call 911.

Schizophrenia And Substance Use Disorders

Substance use disorders occur when frequent use of alcohol and/or drugs interferes with a person's health, family, work, school, and social life. Substance use is the most common co-occurring disorder in people with schizophrenia, and the complex relationships between substance use disorders and schizophrenia have been extensively studied. Substance use disorders can make treatment for schizophrenia less effective, and individuals are also less likely to engage in treatment for their mental illness if they are abusing substances. It is commonly believed that people with schizophrenia who also abuse substances are trying to "self-medicate" their symptoms, but there is little evidence that people begin to abuse substances in response to symptoms or that abusing substances reduces symptoms.

Nicotine is the most common drug abused by people with schizophrenia. People with schizophrenia are much more likely to smoke than people without a mental illness, and researchers are exploring whether there is a biological basis for this. There is some evidence that nicotine may temporarily alleviate a subset of the cognitive deficits commonly observed in schizophrenia, but these benefits are outweighed by the detrimental effects of smoking on other aspects of cognition and general health. Bupropion has been found to be effective for smoking cessation in people with schizophrenia. Most studies find that reducing or stopping smoking does not make schizophrenia symptoms worse.

Cannabis (marijuana) is also frequently abused by people with schizophrenia, which can worsen health outcomes. Heavy cannabis use is associated with more severe and earlier onset of schizophrenia symptoms, but research has not yet definitively determined whether cannabis directly causes schizophrenia.

Drug abuse can increase rates of other medical illnesses (such as hepatitis, heart disease, and infectious disease) as well as suicide, trauma, and homelessness in people with schizophrenia.

It is generally understood that schizophrenia and substance use disorders have strong genetic risk factors. While substance use disorder and a family history of psychosis have individually been identified as risk factors for schizophrenia, it is less well understood if and how these factors are related.

When people have both schizophrenia and a substance abuse disorder, their best chance for recovery is a treatment program that integrates the schizophrenia and substance abuse treatment.

What Causes Schizophrenia?

Research has identified several factors that contribute to the risk of developing schizophrenia.

Genes And Environment

Scientists have long known that schizophrenia sometimes runs in families. The illness occurs in less than 1 percent of the general population, but it occurs in 10 percent of people who have a first-degree relative with the disorder, such as a parent, brother, or sister. People who have second-degree relatives (aunts, uncles, grandparents, or cousins) with the disease also develop schizophrenia more often than the general population. The risk is highest for an identical twin of a person with schizophrenia. He or she has a 40 to 65 percent chance of developing the disorder. Although these genetic relationships are strong, there are many people who have schizophrenia who don't have a family member with the disorder and, conversely, many people with one or more family members with the disorder who do not develop it themselves.

Scientists believe that many different genes contribute to an increased risk of schizophrenia, but that no single gene causes the disorder by itself. In fact, research has found that people with schizophrenia tend to have higher rates of rare genetic mutations. These genetic differences involve hundreds of different genes and probably disrupt brain development in diverse and subtle ways.

Research into various genes that are related to schizophrenia is ongoing, so it is not yet possible to use genetic information to predict who will develop the disease. Despite this, tests that scan a person's genes can be bought without a prescription or a health professional's advice.

Ads for the tests suggest that with a saliva sample, a company can determine if a client is at risk for developing specific diseases, including schizophrenia. However, scientists don't yet know all of the gene variations that contribute to schizophrenia and those that are known raise the risk only by very small amounts. Therefore, these "genome scans" are unlikely to provide a complete picture of a person's risk for developing a mental disorder like schizophrenia.

In addition, it certainly takes more than genes to cause the disorder. Scientists think that interactions between genes and aspects of the individual's environment are necessary for schizophrenia to develop. Many environmental factors may be involved, such as exposure to viruses or malnutrition before birth, problems during birth, and other, not yet known, psychosocial factors.

No one is sure what causes schizophrenia, but your genetic makeup and brain chemistry probably play a role. Medicines can relieve many of the symptoms, but it can take several tries before you find the right drug. You can reduce relapses by staying on your medicine for as long as your doctor recommends. With treatment, many people improve enough to lead satisfying lives.

(Source: "Schizophrenia," MentalHealth.gov, U.S. Department of Health and Human Services (HHS).)

Different Brain Chemistry And Structure

Scientists think that an imbalance in the complex, interrelated chemical reactions of the brain involving the neurotransmitters dopamine and glutamate, and possibly others, plays a role in schizophrenia. Neurotransmitters are substances that brain cells use to communicate with each other. Scientists are learning more about how brain chemistry is related to schizophrenia.

Also, the brain structures of some people with schizophrenia are slightly different than those of healthy people. For example, fluid-filled cavities at the center of the brain, called ventricles, are larger in some people with schizophrenia. The brains of people with the illness also tend to have less gray matter, and some areas of the brain may have less or more activity.

These differences are observed when brain scans from a group of people with schizophrenia are compared with those from a group of people without schizophrenia. However, the differences are not large enough to identify individuals with the disorder and are not currently used to diagnose schizophrenia.

Studies of brain tissue after death also have revealed differences in the brains of people with schizophrenia. Scientists have found small changes in the location or structure of brain cells that are formed before birth. Some experts think problems during brain development before birth may lead to faulty connections. The problem may not show up in a person until puberty. The brain undergoes major changes during puberty, and these changes could trigger psychotic symptoms in people who are vulnerable due to genetics or brain differences. Scientists have learned a lot about schizophrenia, but more research is needed to help explain how it develops.

How Is Schizophrenia Treated?

Because the causes of schizophrenia are still unknown, treatments focus on eliminating the symptoms of the disease. Treatments include antipsychotic medications and various psychosocial treatments. Research on "coordinated specialty care," where a case manager, the patient, and a medication and psychosocial treatment team work together, has shown promising results for recovery.

Antipsychotic Medications

Antipsychotic medications have been available since the mid-1950s. The older types are called conventional or typical antipsychotics.

In the 1990s, new antipsychotic medications were developed. These new medications are called second-generation or atypical antipsychotics.

What Are The Side Effects?

Some people have side effects when they start taking medications. Most side effects go away after a few days. Others are persistent but can often be managed successfully. People who are taking antipsychotic medications should not drive until they adjust to their new medication. Side effects of many antipsychotics include:

- Drowsiness

- Dizziness when changing positions

- Blurred vision

- Rapid heartbeat

- Sensitivity to the sun

- Skin rashes

- Menstrual problems for women

Atypical antipsychotic medications can cause major weight gain and changes in a person's metabolism. This may increase a person's risk of getting diabetes and high cholesterol. A doctor should monitor a person's weight, glucose levels, and lipid levels regularly while the individual is taking an atypical antipsychotic medication.

Typical antipsychotic medications can cause side effects related to physical movement, such as:

- Rigidity

- Persistent muscle spasms

- Tremors

- Restlessness

Doctors and individuals should work together to choose the right medication, medication dose, and treatment plan, which should be based on a person's individual needs and medical situation.

Long-term use of typical antipsychotic medications may lead to a condition called tardive dyskinesia (TD). TD causes muscle movements a person can't control. The movements commonly happen around the mouth. TD can range from mild to severe, and in some people the problem cannot be cured. Sometimes people with TD recover partially or fully after they stop taking the medication.

TD happens to fewer people who take the atypical antipsychotics, but some people may still get TD. People who think that they might have TD should check with their doctor before stopping their medication.

How Are Antipsychotic Medications Taken, And How Do People Respond To Them?

Antipsychotic medications are usually taken daily in pill or liquid form. Some antipsychotics are injections that are given once or twice a month.

Symptoms of schizophrenia, such as feeling agitated and having hallucinations, usually improve within days after starting antipsychotic treatment. Symptoms like delusions usually improve within a few weeks. After about 6 weeks, many people will experience improvement in their symptoms. Some people will continue to have some symptoms, but usually medication helps to keep the symptoms from getting very intense.

However, people respond in different ways to antipsychotic medications, and no one can tell beforehand how a person will respond. Sometimes a person needs to try several medications before finding the right one. Doctors and patients can work together to find the best medication or medication combination, as well as the right dose.

Most people will have one or more periods of relapse—their symptoms come back or get worse. Usually, relapses happen when people stop taking their medication or when they take it less often than prescribed.

Some people stop taking the medication because they feel better or they may feel they don't need it anymore. But no one should stop taking an antipsychotic medication without first talking to his or her doctor. Medication should be gradually tapered off, never stopped suddenly.

How Do Antipsychotic Medications Interact With Other Medications?

Antipsychotic medications can produce unpleasant or dangerous side effects when taken with certain other medications. For this reason, all doctors treating a patient need to be aware of all the medications that person is taking. Doctors need to know about prescription and over-the-counter medicine, vitamins, minerals, and herbal supplements. People also need to discuss any alcohol or street drug use with their doctor.

Psychosocial Treatments

Psychosocial treatments can help people with schizophrenia who are already stabilized. Psychosocial treatments help individuals deal with the everyday challenges of their illness, such as difficulty with communication, work, and forming and keeping relationships. Learning and using coping skills to address these problems helps people with schizophrenia to pursue their life goals, such as attending school or work. Individuals who participate in regular psychosocial treatment are less likely to have relapses or be hospitalized.

Illness Management Skills

People with schizophrenia can take an active role in managing their own illness. Once they learn basic facts about schizophrenia and its treatment, they can make informed decisions about their care. If they know how to watch for the early warning signs of relapse and make a plan to respond, patients can learn to prevent relapses. Patients can also use coping skills to deal with persistent symptoms.

Rehabilitation

Rehabilitation emphasizes social and vocational training to help people with schizophrenia participate fully in their communities. Because the career and life trajectories for individuals with schizophrenia are usually interrupted and they need to learn new skills to get their work life back on track. Rehabilitation programs can include employment services, money management counseling, and skills training to maintain positive relationships.

Family Education And Support

Family education and support teaches relatives or interested individuals about schizophrenia and its treatment and strengthens their capacity to aid in their loved one's recovery.

Cognitive Behavioral Therapy

Cognitive behavioral therapy (CBT) is a type of psychotherapy that focuses on changing unhelpful patterns of thinking and behavior. The CBT therapist teaches people with schizophrenia how to test the reality of their thoughts and perceptions, how to "not listen" to their voices, and how to manage their symptoms overall. CBT can help reduce the severity of symptoms and reduce the risk of relapse. CBT can be delivered individually or in groups.

Self-Help Groups

In self-help groups for people with schizophrenia, group members support and comfort each other and share information on helpful coping strategies and services. Professional therapists usually are not involved. People in self-help groups know that others are facing the same problems, which can help everyone feel less isolated and more connected.

How Can You Help A Person With Schizophrenia?

Family and friends can help their loved one with schizophrenia by supporting their engagement in treatment and pursuit of their recovery goals. Positive communication approaches will be most helpful. It can be difficult to know how to respond to someone with schizophrenia who makes strange or clearly false statements. Remember that these beliefs or hallucinations seem very real to the person. It is not helpful to say they are wrong or imaginary. But going along with the delusions is not helpful, either. Instead, calmly say that you see things differently. Tell them that you acknowledge that everyone has the right to see things his or her own way. In addition, it is important to understand that schizophrenia is a biological illness. Being respectful, supportive, and kind without tolerating dangerous or inappropriate behavior is the best way to approach people with this disorder.

Chapter 16
Borderline Personality Disorder And Suicidality

Borderline personality disorder (BPD) is a serious mental disorder marked by a pattern of ongoing instability in moods, behavior, self-image, and functioning. These experiences often result in impulsive actions and unstable relationships. A person with BPD may experience intense episodes of anger, depression, and anxiety that may last from only a few hours to days.

Some people with BPD also have high rates of co-occurring mental disorders, such as mood disorders, anxiety disorders, and eating disorders, along with substance abuse, self-harm, suicidal thinking and behaviors, and suicide.

While mental health experts now generally agree that the label "borderline personality disorder" is very misleading, a more accurate term does not exist yet.

Signs And Symptoms

People with BPD may experience extreme mood swings and can display uncertainty about who they are. As a result, their interests and values can change rapidly.

Other symptoms include

- frantic efforts to avoid real or imagined abandonment

- a pattern of intense and unstable relationships with family, friends, and loved ones, often swinging from extreme closeness and love (idealization) to extreme dislike or anger (devaluation)

- distorted and unstable self-image or sense of self

About This Chapter: This chapter includes text excerpted from "Borderline Personality Disorder," National Institute of Mental Health (NIMH), August 2016.

- impulsive and often dangerous behaviors, such as spending sprees, unsafe sex, substance abuse, reckless driving, and binge eating

- recurring suicidal behaviors or threats or self-harming behavior, such as cutting

- intense and highly changeable moods, with each episode lasting from a few hours to a few days

- chronic feelings of emptiness

- inappropriate, intense anger or problems controlling anger

- having stress-related paranoid thoughts

- having severe dissociative symptoms, such as feeling cut off from oneself, observing oneself from outside the body, or losing touch with reality

Seemingly ordinary events may trigger symptoms. For example, people with BPD may feel angry and distressed over minor separations—such as vacations, business trips, or sudden changes of plans—from people to whom they feel close. Studies show that people with this disorder may see anger in an emotionally neutral face and have a stronger reaction to words with negative meanings than people who do not have the disorder.

Some of these signs and symptoms may be experienced by people with other mental health problems—and even by people without mental illness—and do not necessarily mean that they have BPD. It is important that a qualified and licensed mental health professional conduct a thorough assessment to determine whether or not a diagnosis of BPD or other mental disorder is warranted, and to help guide treatment options when appropriate.

"Recurrent suicidal behavior, gestures, or threats or self-mutilating behavior" is one of the Diagnostic and Statistical Manual of Mental Disorders (DSM) diagnostic criteria for BPD, and self-injurious behavior has been referred to as the borderline patient's "behavioral specialty." Deliberate self-harm includes suicide attempts (intentionally self-destructive acts accompanied by at least a partial intent to die) and non-suicidal self-harm (intentional self-destructive behavior with no intent to die). It is estimated that as many as 75 percent of patients with BPD make at least one non-lethal suicide attempt, and the rate of actual suicide in patients with BPD is between 8 percent and 10 percent. Risk factors for suicidal behavior in patients with BPD include prior suicide attempts, family history of suicidal behavior, history of sexual abuse, high levels of hopelessness, co-morbid mood disorders and substance use disorders, and high levels of impulsivity and/or antisocial traits.

(Source: "Crossing the Borderline," Agency for Healthcare Research and Quality (AHRQ), U.S. Department of Health and Human Services (HHS).)

Tests And Diagnosis

Unfortunately, BPD is often underdiagnosed or misdiagnosed.

A licensed mental health professional experienced in diagnosing and treating mental disorders—such as a psychiatrist, psychologist, or clinical social worker—can diagnose BPD based on a thorough interview and a comprehensive medical exam, which can help rule out other possible causes of symptoms.

The licensed mental health professional may ask about symptoms and personal and family medical histories, including any history of mental illnesses. This information can help the mental health professional decide on the best treatment. In some cases, co-occurring mental illnesses may have symptoms that overlap with BPD, making it difficult to distinguish BPD from other mental illnesses. For example, a person may describe feelings of depression but may not bring other symptoms to the mental health professional's attention.

Research funded by National Institute of Mental Health (NIMH) is underway to look for ways to improve diagnosis of and treatments for BPD, and to understand the various components of BPD and other personality disorders such as impulsivity, relationship problems, and emotional instability.

Risk Factors

The causes of BPD are not yet clear, but research suggests that genetic, brain, environmental and social factors are likely to be involved.

- **Genetics.** BPD is about five times more likely to occur if a person has a close family member (first-degree biological relatives) with the disorder.

- **Environmental and social factors.** Many people with BPD report experiencing traumatic life events, such as abuse or abandonment during childhood. Others may have been exposed to unstable relationships and hostile conflicts. However, some people with BPD do not have a history of trauma. And, many people with a history of traumatic life events do not have BPD.

- **Brain factors.** Studies show that people with BPD have structural and functional changes in the brain, especially in the areas that control impulses and emotional regulation. However, some people with similar changes in the brain do not have BPD. More research is needed to understand the relationship between brain structure and function and BPD.

Research on BPD is focused on examining biological and environmental risk factors, with special attention on whether early symptoms may emerge at a younger age than previously thought. Scientists are also studying ways to identify the disorder earlier in adolescents.

Treatments And Therapies

BPD has historically been viewed as difficult to treat. However, with newer and proper treatment, many people with BPD experience fewer or less severe symptoms and an improved quality of life. Many factors affect the length of time it takes for symptoms to improve once treatment begins, so it is important for people with BPD and their loved ones to be patient and to receive appropriate support during treatment. People with BPD can recover.

If You Think You Have BPD, It Is Important To Seek Treatment

NIMH-funded studies indicate that BPD patients who never recovered may be more likely to develop other chronic medical conditions and are less likely to make healthy lifestyle choices. BPD is also associated with a high rate of self-harm and suicidal behavior.

> **If you are thinking about harming yourself or attempting suicide, tell someone who can help right away.** Call your licensed mental health professional if you are already working with one. If you are not already working with a licensed mental health professional, call your personal physician or go to the nearest hospital emergency room.
>
> **If a loved one is considering suicide, do not leave him or her alone.** Try to get your loved one to seek immediate help from his or her doctor or the nearest hospital emergency room, or call 911. Remove any access he or she may have to firearms or other potential tools for suicide, including medications, sharp edges such as knives, ropes, or belts.
>
> **If you or a loved one are in crisis:** Call the toll-free National Suicide Prevention Lifeline at 800-273-TALK (800-273-8255), available 24 hours a day, 7 days a week. The service is available to anyone. All calls are confidential.

The treatments described below are just some of the options that may be available to a person with BPD. However, the research on treatments is still in very early stages. More research is needed to determine the effectiveness of these treatments, who may benefit the most, and how best to deliver treatments.

Psychotherapy

Psychotherapy (or "talk therapy") is the main treatment for people with BPD. Current research suggests psychotherapy can relieve some symptoms, but further studies are needed to better understand how well psychotherapy works.

Psychotherapy can be provided one-on-one between the therapist and the patient or in a group setting. Therapist-led group sessions may help teach people with BPD how to interact with others and how to express themselves effectively. It is important that people in therapy get along with and trust their therapist. The very nature of BPD can make it difficult for people with this disorder to maintain a comfortable and trusting bond with their therapist.

Types of psychotherapy used to treat BPD include:

- **Cognitive Behavioral Therapy (CBT):** CBT can help people with BPD identify and change core beliefs and/or behaviors that underlie inaccurate perceptions of themselves and others and problems interacting with others. CBT may help reduce a range of mood and anxiety symptoms and reduce the number of suicidal or self-harming behaviors.

- **Dialectical Behavior Therapy (DBT):** This type of therapy utilizes the concept of mindfulness, or being aware of and attentive to the current situation and moods. DBT also teaches skills to control intense emotions, reduce self-destructive behaviors, and improve relationships. DBT differs from CBT in that it integrates traditional CBT elements with mindfulness, acceptance, and techniques to improve a person's ability to tolerate stress and control his or her emotions. DBT recognizes the dialectical tension between the need for acceptance and the need for change.

- **Schema-Focused Therapy:** This type of therapy combines elements of CBT with other forms of psychotherapy that focus on reframing schemas, or the ways people view themselves. This approach is based on the idea that BPD stems from a dysfunctional self-image—possibly brought on by negative childhood experiences—that affects how people react to their environment, interact with others, and cope with problems or stress.

- **Systems Training for Emotional Predictability and Problem Solving (STEPPS)** is a type of group therapy that aims to educate family members, significant others, and healthcare professionals about BPD and gives them guidance on how to interact consistently with the person with the disorder using the STEPPS approach and terminology. STEPPS is designed to supplement other treatments the patient may be receiving, such as medication or individual psychotherapy.

Families of people with BPD may also benefit from therapy. The challenges of dealing with a loved one with BPD on a daily basis can be very stressful, and family members may unknowingly act in ways that worsen their relative's symptoms. Some therapies include family members in treatment sessions. These types of programs help families develop skills to better understand and support a relative with BPD. Other therapies focus on the needs of family members and help them understand the obstacles and strategies for caring for a loved one with BPD. Although more research is needed to determine the effectiveness of family therapy in BPD, studies on other mental disorders suggest that including family members can help in a person's treatment.

Other types of psychotherapy may be helpful for some people with BPD. Therapists often adapt psychotherapy to better meet a person's needs. Therapists may also switch from one type of psychotherapy to another, mix techniques from different therapies, or use a combination of psychotherapies.

Medications

Medications should not be used as the primary treatment for BPD as the benefits are unclear. However, in some cases, a mental health professional may recommend medications to treat specific symptoms, such as mood swings, depression, or other disorders that may occur with BPD. Treatment with medications may require care from more than one medical professional.

Because of the high risk of suicide among people with BPD, healthcare providers should exercise caution when prescribing medications that may be lethal in the event of an overdose.

Certain medications can cause different side effects in different people. Talk to your doctor about what to expect from a particular medication.

Other Treatments

Some people with BPD experience severe symptoms and require intensive, often inpatient, care. Others may use some outpatient treatments but never need hospitalization or emergency care. Although in rare cases, some people who develop this disorder may improve without any treatment, most people benefit from and improve their quality of life by seeking treatment.

How Can I Help A Friend Or Relative Who Has BPD?

If you know someone who has BPD, it affects you too. The first and most important thing you can do is help your friend or relative get the right diagnosis and treatment. You may need to make an appointment and go with your friend or relative to see the doctor. Encourage him or her to stay in treatment or to seek different treatment if symptoms do not appear to improve with the current treatment.

To help a friend or relative you can:

- Offer emotional support, understanding, patience, and encouragement—change can be difficult and frightening to people with BPD, but it is possible for them to get better over time.

- Learn about mental disorders, including BPD, so you can understand what your friend or relative is experiencing.

- With written permission from your friend or loved one, talk with his or her therapist to learn about therapies that may involve family members. Alternatively, you can encourage your loved one who is in treatment for BPD to ask about family therapy.

- Seek counseling from your own therapist about helping a loved one with BPD. It should not be the same therapist that your loved one with BPD is seeing.

Never ignore comments about someone's intent or plan to harm himself or herself or someone else. Report such comments to the person's therapist or doctor. In urgent or potentially life-threatening situations, you may need to call the police or dial 911.

How Can I Help Myself If I Have BPD?

Although it may take some time, you can get better with treatment. To help yourself:

- Talk to your doctor about treatment options and stick with treatment.

- Try to maintain a stable schedule of meals and sleep times.

- Engage in mild activity or exercise to help reduce stress.

- Set realistic goals for yourself.

- Break up large tasks into small ones, set some priorities, and do what you can, as you can.

- Try to spend time with other people and confide in a trusted friend or family member.

- Tell others about events or situations that may trigger symptoms.

- Expect your symptoms to improve gradually over time, not immediately. Be patient.

- Identify and seek out comforting situations, places, and people.

- Continue to educate yourself about this disorder.

- Don't drink alcohol or use illicit drugs—they will likely make things worse

Borderline Personality Disorder: A Case Study

A 24-year-old woman with BPD was admitted to an inpatient psychiatry unit following a failed suicide attempt with excess doses of acetaminophen. The patient had a history of suicide attempts, including episodes of self-inflicted trauma and abusive behavior. Upon admission, the patient was isolative, displaying a flat affect and expressing a desire to harm herself. When her mood significantly improved after several days of restricted activities, the care team provided her with more freedom, hoping it would improve her condition. Despite occasional gestures suggesting ongoing risk for self-harm as well as continued conflicts with the care team, the patient's behavior became focused on a home visit for her upcoming birthday.

As the care team had observed nearly 72 hours of appropriate behavior, the day before her birthday, they granted permission for the patient's request. Later that evening at home, the patient set herself on fire, prompting immediate return to the hospital for necessary treatment. The events prompted a review and a strengthening of the policies regarding formal risk assessment in this patient population.

The Commentary

BPD is a disorder with an age of onset between 18 and 25. It is categorized in the dramatic/emotional/impulsive cluster of personality disorders; diagnosis is made when five of nine DSM-IV-TR criteria are met, and the prototypic patient with BPD shows a pervasive pattern of instability of mood, impulse control, interpersonal relationships, and self-image. Common comorbidities include mood disorders, anxiety disorders, eating disorders, substance use disorders, other personality disorders, and a range of medical disorders. Some patients electively seek help from a psychiatrist or primary care physician, and they complain of anxiety, depression, or suicidality. Others, feeling distressed by real or perceived maltreatment or rejection by others, may attempt suicide or behave in other self-injurious ways, leading to emergency intervention.

In the case presented here, the patient had known risk factors of former suicide attempts and self-inflicted trauma. It is not clear what precipitated the unsuccessful suicide attempt that led to the current hospitalization, but clarifying the interpersonal circumstances that were occurring in her life prior to the suicide attempt would be crucial. Patients with BPD frequently demonstrate mood shifts, and this patient, in the structured setting of the hospital, shed her dysphoria and requested a home visit for her birthday. Who was at home? What was the nature of the patient's relationships with those at home? What have previous birthday celebrations been like? Since family stress and interpersonal conflicts are so common for patients with BPD, birthdays are often formulas for disappointment. In this case, perhaps all signals were green and the self-injury on the home visit could not have been anticipated. However, given the modal pattern of disturbed family and interpersonal relationships for patients with BPD, it seems far more likely that the patient's expectation of a positive home visit on her birthday represented an idealized fantasy. Patients with BPD can become angry and oppositional when challenged, and the staff may have supported the patient's request partially, at least, to prevent a regressive eruption of rage and the possibility of reactivated self-injurious behavior in the hospital.

(Source: "Crossing the Borderline," Agency for Healthcare Research and Quality (AHRQ), U.S. Department of Health and Human Services (HHS).)

Chapter 17
Abuse Of Alcohol And Other Substances Increases Suicide Risk

Basic Facts About Substance Abuse

- Suicide is a leading cause of death among people who abuse alcohol and drugs.

- Compared to the general population, individuals treated for alcohol abuse or dependence are at about 10 times greater risk to eventually die by suicide compared with the general population, and people who inject drugs are at about 14 times greater risk for eventual suicide.

- Individuals with substance use disorders are also at elevated risk for suicidal ideation and suicide attempts.

- People with substance use disorders who are in treatment are at especially high risk of suicidal behavior for many reasons, including:

- They enter treatment at a point when their substance abuse is out of control, increasing a variety of risk factors for suicide.

- They enter treatment when a number of co-occurring life crises may be occurring (e.g., marital, legal, job).

- They enter treatment at peaks in depressive symptoms.

- Mental health problems (e.g., depression, posttraumatic stress disorder (PTSD), anxiety disorders, some personality disorders) associated with suicidality often co-occur among people who have been treated for substance use disorders.

About This Chapter: This chapter includes text excerpted from "Addressing Suicidal Thoughts And Behaviors In Substance Abuse Treatment," Substance Abuse and Mental Health Services Administration (SAMHSA), 2015.

- Crises that are known to increase suicide risk sometimes occur during treatment (e.g., relapse and treatment transitions).

LGBT Youth And Substance Abuse

LGBT youth may be more likely to use substances to cope with bias and stress and may be more likely to experience increased rates of depression and anxiety than their non-LGBT peers. Challenges such as family rejection of, or anticipated reaction to, one's LGBT identity are also associated with substance use. For example, one study found that youth who experienced a moderate level of family rejection were 1.5 times more likely to use illegal substances than those who experienced little to no rejection; youth experiencing high levels of family rejection were 3.5 times more likely to use these substances. Also, youth who have run away from home have higher rates of alcohol and illicit drug use.

(Source: "LGBT: Behavioral Health," Youth.gov.)

The Link Between Substance Abuse And Suicidality

There is a strong link between substance use disorders and risk for suicidal behavior.

- Suicide is a leading cause of death among people who abuse alcohol and drugs.

- Compared with the general population, individuals treated for alcohol abuse or dependence are at about 10 times greater risk for suicide; people who inject drugs are at about 14 times greater risk for suicide.

- Individuals with substance use disorders are also at increased risk for suicidal ideation and suicide attempts.

- Depression is a common co-occurring diagnosis among people who abuse substances that confers risk for suicidal behavior. Other mental disorders are also implicated.

- People with substance use disorders often seek treatment at times when their substance use difficulties are at their peak—a vulnerable period that may be accompanied by suicidal thoughts and behaviors.

There is a strong link between acute substance use and risk for suicidal behavior.

- Alcohol's acute effects include disinhibition, intense focus on the current situation with little appreciation for consequences, and promoting depressed mood, all of which may increase risk for suicidal behavior. Other central nervous system depressants may act similarly.

- Acute alcohol intoxication is present in about 30–40 percent of suicide attempts and suicides.

- Intense, short-lived depression is prevalent among treatment-seeking people who abuse cocaine, methamphetamines, and alcohol, among other groups. Even transient depression is a potent risk factor for suicidal behavior among people with substance use disorders.

- Overdose suicides often involve multiple drugs like alcohol, benzodiazepines, opioids, and other psychiatric medications.

The risk for suicidal behavior may increase at any point in treatment.

- Suicide risk may increase at transition points in care (inpatient to outpatient, intensive treatment to continuing care, discharge), especially when a planned transition breaks down. Anticipating risk at such transition points should be regarded as an issue in treatment planning.

- Suicide risk may increase when a client is terminated administratively (e.g., because of poor attendance, chronic substance use) or is refused care. It is unethical to discharge a client and/or refuse care to someone who is suicidal without making appropriate alternative arrangements for treatment to address suicide risk.

- Suicide risk may increase in clients with a history of suicidal thoughts or attempts who relapse. Treatment plans for such clients should provide for this possibility.

- Suicide risk may increase in clients with a history of suicidal thoughts or attempts who imply that the worst might happen if they relapse (e.g., "I can't go through this again," "if I relapse, that's it")—especially for those who make a direct threat (e.g., "This is my last chance; if I relapse, I'm going to kill myself"). Treatment plans for such clients should provide for this possibility.

- Suicide risk may increase in clients with a history of suicidal thoughts or attempts when they are experiencing acute stressful life events. Treatment plans for such clients should provide for this possibility, for example, by adding more intensive treatment, closer observation, or additional services to manage the life crises.

The Link Between Marijuana Use And Psychiatric Disorders

Several studies have linked marijuana use to increased risk for psychiatric disorders, including psychosis (schizophrenia), depression, anxiety, and substance use disorders, but whether and to what extent it actually causes these conditions is not always easy to determine. The amount of drug used, the age at first use, and genetic vulnerability have all been shown to influence this relationship. The strongest evidence to date concerns links between marijuana use and substance use disorders and between marijuana use and psychiatric disorders in those with a preexisting genetic or other vulnerability.

(Source: "Is There A Link Between Marijuana Use And Psychiatric Disorders?" National Institute on Drug Abuse (NIDA).)

Chapter 18
Abusing Prescription And Over-The-Counter (OTC) Drugs

The Abuse Of Prescription Medication

Some medications have psychoactive (mind-altering) properties and, because of that, are sometimes abused—that is, taken for reasons or in ways or amounts not intended by a doctor, or taken by someone other than the person for whom they are prescribed. In fact, prescription and over-the-counter (OTC) drugs are, after marijuana (and alcohol), the most commonly abused substances by Americans 14 and older.

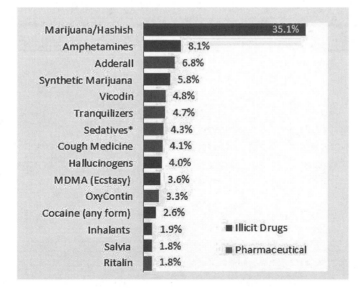

Figure 18.1. Past-Year Use Of Various Drugs By 12th Graders (Percent)

About This Chapter: This chapter includes text excerpted from "DrugFacts—Prescription And Over-The-Counter Medications," National Institute on Drug Abuse (NIDA), November 2015.

The classes of prescription drugs most commonly abused are: opioid pain relievers, such as Vicodin® or Oxycontin®; stimulants for treating attention deficit hyperactivity disorder (ADHD), such as Adderall®, Concerta®, or Ritalin®; and central nervous system (CNS) depressants for relieving anxiety, such as Valium® or Xanax®. The most commonly abused OTC drugs are cough and cold remedies containing dextromethorphan.

People often think that prescription and OTC drugs are safer than illicit drugs. But they can be as addictive and dangerous and put users at risk for other adverse health effects, including overdose—especially when taken along with other drugs or alcohol. Before prescribing drugs, a healthcare provider considers a patient's health conditions, current and prior drug use, and other medicines to assess the risks and benefits for a patient.

How Are Prescription Drugs Abused?

Prescription and OTC drugs may be abused in one or more of the following ways:

Taking a medication that has been prescribed for somebody else. Unaware of the dangers of sharing medications, people often unknowingly contribute to this form of abuse by sharing their unused pain relievers with their family members.

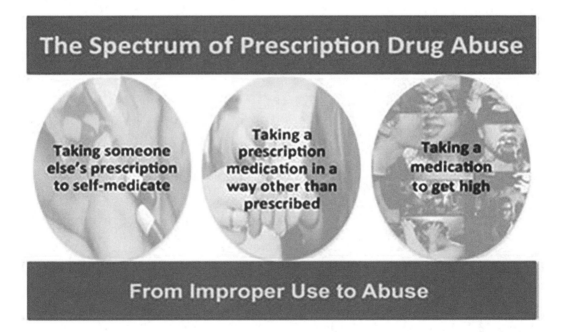

Figure 18.2. Spectrum Of Prescription Drug Abuse

Most teenagers who abuse prescription drugs are given them for free by a friend or relative.

Taking a drug in a higher quantity or in another manner than prescribed. Most prescription drugs are dispensed orally in tablets, but abusers sometimes crush the tablets and snort or inject the powder. This hastens the entry of the drug into the bloodstream and the brain and amplifies its effects.

Taking a drug for another purpose than prescribed. All of the drug types mentioned can produce pleasurable effects at sufficient quantities, so taking them for the purpose of getting high is one of the main reasons people abuse them.

ADHD drugs like Adderall® are also often abused by students seeking to improve their academic performance. However, although they may boost alertness, there is little evidence they improve cognitive functioning for those without a medical condition.

How Do Prescription And OTC Drugs Affect The Brain?

Taken as intended, prescription and OTC drugs safely treat specific mental or physical symptoms. But when taken in different quantities or when such symptoms aren't present, they may affect the brain in ways very similar to illicit drugs.

For example, stimulants such as Ritalin® achieve their effects by acting on the same neurotransmitter systems as cocaine. Opioid pain relievers such as OxyContin® attach to the same cell receptors targeted by illegal opioids like heroin. Prescription depressants produce sedating or calming effects in the same manner as the club drugs GHB and Rohypnol®. And when taken in very high doses, dextromethorphan acts on the same cell receptors as PCP or ketamine, producing similar out-of-body experiences.

When abused, all of these classes of drugs directly or indirectly cause a pleasurable increase in the amount of dopamine in the brain's reward pathway. Repeatedly seeking to experience that feeling can lead to addiction.

What Are The Other Health Effects Of Prescription And OTC Drugs?

Opioids can produce drowsiness, cause constipation, and—depending upon the amount taken—depress breathing. The latter effect makes opioids particularly dangerous, especially when they are snorted or injected or combined with other drugs or alcohol.

Opioids And Brain Damage

While the relationship between opioid overdose and depressed respiration (slowed breathing) has been confirmed, researchers are also studying the long-term effects on brain function. Depressed respiration can affect the amount of oxygen that reaches the brain, a condition called hypoxia. Hypoxia can have short- and long-term psychological and neurological effects, including coma and permanent brain damage.

Researchers are also investigating the long-term effects of opioid addiction on the brain. Studies have shown some deterioration of the brain's white matter due to heroin use, which may affect decision-making abilities, the ability to regulate behavior, and responses to stressful situations.

More people die from overdoses of prescription opioids than from all other drugs combined, including heroin and cocaine.

The Prescription Opioid Overdose Epidemic

More than 2 million people in the United States suffer from substance use disorders related to prescription opioid pain relievers. The terrible consequences of this trend include overdose deaths, which have more than quadrupled in the past decade and a half. The causes are complex, but they include overprescription of pain medications. In 2013, 207 million prescriptions were written for prescription opioid pain medications.

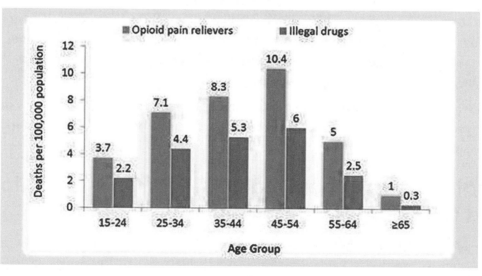

Figure 18.3. Deaths From Opioid Pain Relievers Exceed Those From All Illegal Drugs

Stimulants can have strong effects on the cardiovascular system. Taking high doses of a stimulant can dangerously raise body temperature and cause irregular heartbeat or even heart failure or seizures. Also, taking some stimulants in high doses or repeatedly can lead to hostility or feelings of paranoia.

CNS depressants slow down brain activity and can cause sleepiness and loss of coordination. Continued use can lead to physical dependence and withdrawal symptoms if discontinuing use.

Dextromethorphan can cause impaired motor function, numbness, nausea or vomiting, and increased heart rate and blood pressure. On rare occasions, hypoxic brain damage—caused by severe respiratory depression and a lack of oxygen to the brain—has occurred due to the combination of dextromethorphan with decongestants often found in the medication.

All of these drugs have the potential for addiction, and this risk is amplified when they are abused. Also, as with other drugs, abuse of prescription and OTC drugs can alter a person's judgment and decision making, leading to dangerous behaviors such as unsafe sex and drugged driving.

Prescription Opioid Abuse: A First Step To Heroin Use?

Prescription opioid pain medications such as Oxycontin® and Vicodin® can have effects similar to heroin when taken in doses or in ways other than prescribed, and research now suggests that abuse of these drugs may actually open the door to heroin abuse.

Nearly half of young people who inject heroin surveyed in three studies reported abusing prescription opioids before starting to use heroin. Some individuals reported taking up heroin because it is cheaper and easier to obtain than prescription opioids.

Many of these young people also report that crushing prescription opioid pills to snort or inject the powder provided their initiation into these methods of drug administration.

Chapter 19
Abusive Relationships May Increase Suicide Risk

Teen Dating Violence

Dating violence is a type of intimate partner violence. It occurs between two people in a close relationship. The nature of dating violence can be physical, emotional, or sexual.

- **Physical**—This occurs when a partner is pinched, hit, shoved, slapped, punched, or kicked.

- **Psychological/Emotional**—This means threatening a partner or harming his or her sense of self-worth. Examples include name calling, shaming, bullying, embarrassing on purpose, or keeping him/her away from friends and family.

- **Sexual**—This is forcing a partner to engage in a sex act when he or she does not or cannot consent. This can be physical or nonphysical, like threatening to spread rumors if a partner refuses to have sex.

- **Stalking**—This refers to a pattern of harassing or threatening tactics that are unwanted and cause fear in the victim.

Dating violence can take place in person or electronically, such as repeated texting or posting sexual pictures of a partner online.

Unhealthy relationships can start early and last a lifetime. Teens often think some behaviors, like teasing and name calling, are a "normal" part of a relationship. However, these behaviors can become abusive and develop into more serious forms of violence.

About This Chapter: Text under the heading "Teen Dating Violence" is excerpted from "Understanding Teen Dating Violence," Centers for Disease Control and Prevention (CDC), 2016; Text under the heading "Child Abuse" is excerpted from "Child Abuse Leaves Epigenetic Marks," National Human Genome Research Institute (NHGRI), July 3, 2013. Reviewed January 2017.

Why Is Dating Violence A Public Health Problem?

Dating violence is a widespread issue that has serious long-term and short-term effects. Many teens do not report it because they are afraid to tell friends and family.

Among high school students who dated, 21 percent of females and 10 percent of males experienced physical and/ or sexual dating violence.

Among adult victims of rape, physical violence, and/ or stalking by an intimate partner, 22 percent of women and 15 percent of men first experienced some form of partner violence between 11 and 17 years of age.

How Does Dating Violence Affect Health?

Dating violence can have a negative effect on health throughout life. Youth who are victims are more likely to experience symptoms of depression and anxiety, engage in unhealthy behaviors, like using tobacco, drugs, and alcohol, or exhibit antisocial behaviors and think about suicide. Youth who are victims of dating violence in high school are at higher risk for victimization during college.

Who Is At Risk For Dating Violence?

Factors that increase risk for harming a dating partner include the following:

- belief that dating violence is acceptable
- depression, anxiety, and other trauma symptoms
- aggression towards peers and other aggressive behavior
- substance use
- early sexual activity and having multiple sexual partners
- having a friend involved in dating violence
- conflict with partner
- witnessing or experiencing violence in the home

How Can We Prevent Dating Violence?

The ultimate goal is to stop dating violence before it starts. Strategies that promote healthy relationships are vital. During the preteen and teen years, young people are learning skills they need to form positive relationships with others. This is an ideal time to promote healthy relationships and prevent patterns of dating violence that can last into adulthood.

Many prevention strategies are proven to prevent or reduce dating violence. Some effective school-based programs change norms, improve problem-solving, and address dating violence in addition to other youth risk behaviors, such as substance use and sexual risk behaviors. Other programs prevent dating violence through changes to the school environment or training influential adults, like parents/caregivers and coaches, to work with youth to prevent dating violence.

Child Abuse

Child abuse is a serious national and global problem that cuts across economic, racial and cultural lines. Each year, more than 1.25 million children are abused or neglected in the United States, with that number expanding to at least 40 million per year worldwide.

In addition to harming the immediate well-being of the child, maltreatment and extreme stress during childhood can impair early brain development and metabolic and immune system function, leading to chronic health problems. As a consequence, abused children are at increased risk for a wide range of physical health conditions including obesity, heart disease, and cancer, as well as psychiatric conditions such as depression, suicide, drug and alcohol abuse, high-risk behaviors and violence.

They are also more susceptible to developing posttraumatic stress disorder (PTSD)—a severe and debilitating stress-related psychiatric disorder-after experiencing other types of trauma later in life.

Part of the explanation is that child abuse can leave marks, not only physically and emotionally, but also in the form of epigenetic marks on a child's genes. Although these epigenetic marks do not cause mutations in the DNA itself, the chemical modifications—including DNA methylation—change gene expression by silencing (or activating) genes. This can alter fundamental biological processes and adversely affect health outcomes throughout life.

Chapter 20
Self-Injury In Teens

What Is Self-Injury?

Self-harm, sometimes called self-injury, is when a person purposely hurts his or her own body. There are many types of self-injury, and cutting is one type that you may have heard about. If you are hurting yourself, you can learn to stop. Make sure you talk to an adult you trust, and keep reading to learn more.

What Are Ways People Hurt Themselves?

Some types of injury leave permanent scars or cause serious health problems, sometimes even death. These are some forms of self-injury:

- Cutting yourself (such as using a razorblade, knife, or other sharp object)

- Punching yourself or punching things (like a wall)

- Burning yourself with cigarettes, matches, or candles

- Pulling out your hair

- Poking objects into body openings

- Breaking your bones or bruising yourself

- Poisoning yourself

About This Chapter: This chapter includes text excerpted from "Cutting And Self-Harm," girlshealth.gov, Office on Women's Health (OWH), January 7, 2015.

The Dangers Of Self-Injury

Some teens think self-injury is not a big deal, but it is. Self-injury comes with many risks. For example, cutting can lead to infections, scars, and even death. Sharing tools for cutting puts a person at risk of diseases like HIV and hepatitis. Also, once you start self-injuring, it may be hard to stop. And teens who keep hurting themselves are less likely to learn how to deal with their feelings in healthy ways.

Who Hurts Themselves?

People from all different kinds of backgrounds hurt themselves. Among teens, girls may be more likely to do it than boys.

People of all ages hurt themselves, too, but self-injury most often starts in the teen years.

People who hurt themselves sometimes have other problems like depression, eating disorders, or drug or alcohol abuse.

> ## Children And Youth With Disabilities
> Children and youth with developmental disabilities, such as autism and intellectual disability, are more likely to engage in other forms of self-injury than children without these disabilities. Youth with depression, anxiety disorder, and conduct disorder have a higher chance of self-violence, including suicide, than children without these disorders.
>
> *(Source: "Safety And Children With Disabilities: Self Injury," National Center on Birth Defects and Developmental Disabilities (NCBDDD), Centers for Disease Control and Prevention (CDC).)*

Why Do Some Teens Hurt Themselves?

Some teens who hurt themselves keep their feelings bottled up inside. The physical pain then offers a sense of relief, like the feelings are getting out. Some people who hold back strong emotions begin to feel like they have no emotions, and the injury helps them at least feel something.

Some teens say that when they hurt themselves, they are trying to stop feeling painful emotions, like rage, loneliness, or hopelessness. They may injure to distract themselves from the emotional pain. Or they may be trying to feel some sense of control over what they feel.

If you are depressed, angry, or having a hard time coping, talk with an adult you trust. You also can contact a helpline. Remember, you have a right to be safe and happy!

If you are hurting yourself, please get help. It is possible to get past the urge to hurt yourself. There are other ways to deal with your feelings. You can talk to your parents, your doctor, or another trusted adult, like a teacher or religious leader. Therapy can help you find healthy ways to handle problems.

Those who self-harm very often have a history of childhood sexual abuse. For example, in one group of self-harmers, 93 percent said they had been sexually abused in childhood. Some research has looked at whether certain aspects of childhood sexual abuse increase the risk that survivors will engage in self-harm as adults. The findings show that more severe, more frequent, or longer-lasting sexual abuse is linked to an increased risk of engaging in self-harm in one's adult years.

(Source: "Self-Harm And Trauma," National Center for Posttraumatic Stress Disorder (NCPTSD), U.S. Department of Veterans Affairs (VA).)

What Are Signs Of Self-Injury In Others?

- Having cuts, bruises, or scars
- Wearing long sleeves or pants even in hot weather
- Making excuses about injuries
- Having sharp objects around for no clear reason

How Can I Help A Friend Who Is Self-Injuring?

If you think a friend may be hurting herself, try to get your friend to talk to a trusted adult. Your friend may need professional help. A therapist can suggest ways to cope with problems without turning to self-injury. If your friend won't get help, you should talk to an adult. This is too much for you to handle alone.

What If Someone Pressures Me To Hurt Myself?

If someone pressures you to hurt yourself, think about whether you really want a friend who tries to cause you pain. Try to hang out with other people who don't treat you this way. Try to hang out with people who make you feel good about yourself.

Chapter 21
Eating Disorders

Eating Disorders And Suicidal Thoughts

What is the most fatal mental disorder? The answer, which may surprise you, is anorexia nervosa. It has an estimated mortality rate of around 10 percent. What is the cause of this high rate of mortality? The answer is complicated. While many young women and men with this disorder die from starvation and metabolic collapse, others die of suicide, which is much more common in women with anorexia than most other mental disorders.

> People with eating disorders are more likely to think about suicide. If you or someone you know is thinking about suicide, get help. You can call the suicide hotline at 800-273-TALK (800-273-8255) or 911 for immediate help.
>
> *(Source: "Having Eating Disorders," girlshealth.gov, Office on Women's Health (OWH).)*

What Are Eating Disorders?

There is a commonly held view that eating disorders are a lifestyle choice. Eating disorders are actually serious and often fatal illnesses that cause severe disturbances to a person's eating behaviors. Obsessions with food, body weight, and shape may also signal an eating disorder. Common eating disorders include anorexia nervosa, bulimia nervosa, and binge eating disorder.

About This Chapter: Text under the heading "Eating Disorders And Suicidal Thoughts" is excerpted from "Post By Former NIMH Director Thomas Insel: Spotlight On Eating Disorders," National Institute of Mental Health (NIMH), February 24, 2012. Reviewed January 2017; Text beginning with the heading "What Are Eating Disorders?" is excerpted from "Eating Disorders," National Institute of Mental Health (NIMH), February 2016.

Signs And Symptoms

Anorexia Nervosa

People with anorexia nervosa may see themselves as overweight, even when they are dangerously underweight. People with anorexia nervosa typically weigh themselves repeatedly, severely restrict the amount of food they eat, and eat very small quantities of only certain foods. Anorexia nervosa has the highest mortality rate of any mental disorder. While many young women and men with this disorder die from complications associated with starvation, others die of suicide. In women, suicide is much more common in those with anorexia than with most other mental disorders.

Symptoms include:

• Extremely restricted eating

• Extreme thinness (emaciation)

• A relentless pursuit of thinness and unwillingness to maintain a normal or healthy weight

• Intense fear of gaining weight

• Distorted body image, a self-esteem that is heavily influenced by perceptions of body weight and shape, or a denial of the seriousness of low body weight

Other symptoms may develop over time, including:

• Thinning of the bones (osteopenia or osteoporosis)

• Mild anemia and muscle wasting and weakness

• Brittle hair and nails

• Dry and yellowish skin

• Growth of fine hair all over the body (lanugo)

• Severe constipation

• Low blood pressure, slowed breathing and pulse

• Damage to the structure and function of the heart

• Brain damage

• Multiorgan failure

- Drop in internal body temperature, causing a person to feel cold all the time

- Lethargy, sluggishness, or feeling tired all the time

- Infertility

Bulimia Nervosa

People with bulimia nervosa have recurrent and frequent episodes of eating unusually large amounts of food and feeling a lack of control over these episodes. This binge eating is followed by behavior that compensates for the overeating such as forced vomiting, excessive use of laxatives or diuretics, fasting, excessive exercise, or a combination of these behaviors. Unlike anorexia nervosa, people with bulimia nervosa usually maintain what is considered a healthy or relatively normal weight.

Symptoms include:

- Chronically inflamed and sore throat

- Swollen salivary glands in the neck and jaw area

- Worn tooth enamel and increasingly sensitive and decaying teeth as a result of exposure to stomach acid

- Acid reflux disorder and other gastrointestinal problems

- Intestinal distress and irritation from laxative abuse

- Severe dehydration from purging of fluids

- Electrolyte imbalance (too low or too high levels of sodium, calcium, potassium and other minerals) which can lead to stroke or heart attack

In research supported by the National Institute of Mental Health (NIMH), scientists have found that many patients with anorexia also suffer from psychiatric illnesses. While the majority have co-occurring clinical depression, others suffer from anxiety, personality, or substance abuse disorders, and many are at risk for suicide. Obsessive compulsive disorder (OCD), an illness characterized by repetitive thoughts and behaviors, can also accompany anorexia. Individuals with anorexia are typically compliant in personality but may have sudden outbursts of hostility and anger or become socially withdrawn.

Some individuals with bulimia struggle with addictions, including abuse of drugs and alcohol, and compulsive stealing. Like individuals with anorexia, many people with bulimia suffer from clinical depression, anxiety, OCD, and other psychiatric illnesses. These problems, combined with their impulsive tendencies, place them at increased risk for suicidal behavior.

(Source: "Providing Support For Suicide Survivors: Understanding Pertinent Military/Veteran Issues," U.S. Department of Commerce (DOC), Western Region Security Office (WRSO).)

Binge Eating Disorder

People with binge eating disorder lose control over his or her eating. Unlike bulimia nervosa, periods of binge eating are not followed by purging, excessive exercise, or fasting. As a result, people with binge eating disorder often are overweight or obese. Binge eating disorder is the most common eating disorder in the United States.

Symptoms include:

- Eating unusually large amounts of food in a specific amount of time

- Eating even when you're full or not hungry

- Eating fast during binge episodes

- Eating until you're uncomfortably full

- Eating alone or in secret to avoid embarrassment

- Feeling distressed, ashamed, or guilty about your eating

- Frequently dieting, possibly without weight loss

Risk Factors

Eating disorders frequently appear during the teen years or young adulthood but may also develop during childhood or later in life. These disorders affect both genders, although rates among women are 2½ times greater than among men. Like women who have eating disorders, men also have a distorted sense of body image. For example, men may have muscle dysmorphia, a type of disorder marked by an extreme concern with becoming more muscular.

Researchers are finding that eating disorders are caused by a complex interaction of genetic, biological, behavioral, psychological, and social factors. Researchers are using the latest technology and science to better understand eating disorders.

One approach involves the study of human genes. Eating disorders run in families. Researchers are working to identify DNA variations that are linked to the increased risk of developing eating disorders.

Brain imaging studies are also providing a better understanding of eating disorders. For example, researchers have found differences in patterns of brain activity in women with eating disorders in comparison with healthy women. This kind of research can help guide the development of new means of diagnosis and treatment of eating disorders.

Treatments And Therapies

Adequate nutrition, reducing excessive exercise, and stopping purging behaviors are the foundations of treatment. Treatment plans are tailored to individual needs and may include one or more of the following:

- Individual, group, and/or family psychotherapy
- Medical care and monitoring
- Nutritional counseling
- Medications

Psychotherapies

Psychotherapies such as a family-based therapy called the Maudsley approach, where parents of adolescents with anorexia nervosa assume responsibility for feeding their child, appear to be very effective in helping people gain weight and improve eating habits and moods.

To reduce or eliminate binge eating and purging behaviors, people may undergo cognitive behavioral therapy (CBT), which is another type of psychotherapy that helps a person learn how to identify distorted or unhelpful thinking patterns and recognize and change inaccurate beliefs.

Medications

Evidence also suggests that medications such as antidepressants, antipsychotics, or mood stabilizers approved by the U.S. Food and Drug Administration (FDA) may also be helpful for treating eating disorders and other co-occurring illnesses such as anxiety or depression.

Chapter 22
Bullying And Suicide

What We Know About Bullying And Suicide

In the past decade, headlines reporting the tragic stories of a young person's suicide death linked in some way to bullying (physical, verbal, or online) have become regrettably common. There is so much pain and suffering associated with each of these events, affecting individuals, families, communities and our society as a whole and resulting in an increasing national outcry to "do something" about the problem of bullying and suicide.

For this reason, the Centers for Disease Control and Prevention (CDC) and other violence prevention partners and researchers have invested in learning more about the relationship between these two serious public health problems with the goal of using this knowledge to save lives and prevent future bullying.

Bullying

- Bullying is unwanted, aggressive behavior among school-aged children that involves a real or perceived power imbalance. The behavior is repeated, or has the potential to be repeated, over time. Bullying includes actions such as making threats, spreading rumors, attacking someone physically or verbally, and excluding someone from a group on purpose. Bullying can occur in-person or through technology.

- Bullying has serious and lasting negative effects on the mental health and overall well-being of youth involved in bullying in any way including: those who bully others, youth

About This Chapter: This chapter includes text excerpted from "The Relationship Between Bullying And Suicide: What We Know And What It Means For Schools," Centers for Disease Control and Prevention (CDC), April 2014.

who are bullied, as well as those youth who both bully others and are bullied by others, sometimes referred to as bully-victims.

- Even youth who have observed but not participated in bullying behavior report significantly more feelings of helplessness and less sense of connectedness and support from responsible adults (parents/schools) than youth who are have not witnessed bullying behavior.

- Negative outcomes of bullying (for youth who bully others, youth who are bullied, and youth who both are bullied and bully others) may include: depression, anxiety, involvement in interpersonal violence or sexual violence, substance abuse, poor social functioning, and poor school performance, including lower grade point averages, standardized test scores, and poor attendance.

- Youth who report frequently bullying others and youth who report being frequently bullied are at increased risk for suicide-related behavior.

- Youth who report both bullying others and being bullied (bully-victims) have the highest risk for suicide-related behavior of any groups that report involvement in bullying.

Suicide

- Suicide-related behaviors include the following:

  - **Suicide:** Death caused by self-directed injurious behavior with any intent to die.

  - **Suicide attempt:** A non-fatal self-directed potentially injurious behavior with any intent to die as a result of the behavior. A suicide attempt may or may not result in injury.

  - **Suicidal ideation:** Thinking about, considering, or planning for suicide.

- Suicide-related behavior is complicated and rarely the result of a single source of trauma or stress.

- People who engage in suicide-related behavior often experience overwhelming feelings of helplessness and hopelessness.

- ANY involvement with bullying behavior is one stressor which may significantly contribute to feelings of helplessness and hopelessness that raise the risk of suicide.

- Youth who are at increased risk for suicide-related behavior are dealing with a complex interaction of multiple relationship (peer, family, or romantic), mental health, and school stressors.

What We Know About Bullying And Suicide Together

- We know that bullying behavior and suicide-related behavior are closely related. This means youth who report any involvement with bullying behavior are more likely to report high levels of suicide-related behavior than youth who do not report any involvement with bullying behavior.

- We know enough about the relationship between bullying and suicide-related behavior to make evidence-based recommendations to improve prevention efforts.

What We DON'T Know About Bullying And Suicide

We don't know if bullying directly causes suicide-related behavior. We know that most youth who are involved in bullying do NOT engage in suicide-related behavior. It is correct to say that involvement in bullying, along with other risk factors, increases the chance that a young person will engage in suicide-related behaviors.

The Relationship Between Bullying And Suicide

Recent attention focused on the relationship between bullying and suicide is positive and helpful because it:

- Raises awareness about the serious harm that bullying does to all youth involved in bullying in any way.

- Highlights the significant risk for our most vulnerable youth (e.g., youth with disabilities, youth with learning differences, LGBTQ youth).

- Encourages conversation about the problem of bullying and suicide and promotes collaboration around prevention locally and nationally.

However, framing the discussion of the issue as bullying being a single, direct cause of suicide is not helpful and is potentially harmful because it could:

1. Perpetuate the false notion that suicide is a natural response to being bullied which has the dangerous potential to normalize the response and thus create copycat behavior among youth.

2. Encourage sensationalized reporting and contradicts the Recommendations for Reporting on Suicide (reportingonsuicide.org) potentially encouraging copycat behavior that could lead to "suicide contagion."

3. Focus the response on blame and punishment which misdirects the attention from getting the needed support and treatment to those who are bullied as well as those who bully others.

4. Take attention away from other important risk factors for suicidal behavior that need to be addressed (e.g., substance abuse, mental illnesses, problems coping with disease/disability, family dysfunction, etc.)

Still, a report of a young person who takes his/her own life and leaves a note pointing directly to the suffering and pain they have endured because of bullying is shocking and heart-breaking. While a young person's death by suicide is a tragedy and both bullying and suicide-related behavior are serious public health problems, our response to such situations must reflect a balanced understanding of the issues informed by the best available research.

It is particularly important to understand the difference between circumstances being related to an event versus being direct causes or effects of the event. To explore this idea, let's look at a similar but much simpler example:

In the case of drowning deaths among children, those who are not directly supervised by a competent adult while swimming are more likely to die by drowning than those children who are directly supervised. While the lack of adult supervision does not directly cause a child to drown, it is a critical circumstance that can affect the outcome of the situation.

Just as with preventing deaths by drowning, for bullying and suicide prevention, the more we understand about the relationship between circumstances and outcomes the better decisions we can make about what actions to take to prevent bullying and suicide-related behavior.

So, if bullying doesn't directly cause suicide, what do we know about how bullying and suicide are related?

Bullying and suicide-related behavior are both complex public health problems. Circumstances that can affect a person's vulnerability to either or both of these behaviors exist at a variety of levels of influence—individual, family, community, and society. These include:

• emotional distress

• exposure to violence

• family conflict

• relationship problems

• lack of connectedness to school/sense of supportive school environment

- alcohol and drug use

- physical disabilities/learning differences

- lack of access to resources/support.

If, however, students experience the opposite of some of the circumstances listed above (e.g., family support rather than family conflict; strong school connectedness rather than lack of connectedness), their risk for suicide-related behavior and/or bullying others—even if they experience bullying behavior—might be reduced. These types of circumstances/situations or behaviors are sometimes referred to as "protective factors."

In reality, most students have a combination of risk and protective factors for bullying behavior and suicide-related behavior. This is one of the reasons that we emphasize that the relationship between the two behaviors and their health outcomes is not simple. The ultimate goal of our prevention efforts is to reduce risk factors and increase protective factors as much as possiblc.

The bottom-line of the most current research findings is that being involved in bullying in any way—as a person who bullies, a person who is bullied, or a person who both bullies and is bullied (bully-victim)—is ONE of several important risk factors that appears to increase the risk of suicide among youth.

What Can We Do With What We Know?

Knowledge is really most helpful if it informs action toward a positive change—in this case, prevention of bullying and suicide-related behavior. The following paragraph highlights key research findings about the relationship between bullying and suicide-related behavior.

What Do We Know From Research?

- Youth who feel connected to their school are less likely to engage in suicide-related behaviors.

- Youth who are able to cope with problems in healthy ways and solve problems peacefully are less likely to engage in suicide and bullying related behaviors.

- Youth with disabilities, learning differences, sexual/gender identity differences or cultural differences are often most vulnerable to being bullied.

- Youth who report frequently bullying others are at high, long-term risk for suicide-related behavior.

- Youth who report both being bullied and bullying others (sometimes referred to as bully-victims) have the highest rates of negative mental health outcomes, including depression, anxiety, and thinking about suicide.

- Youth who report being frequently bullied by others are at increased risk of suicide-related behaviors, and negative physical and mental health outcomes.

- Involvement in bullying in any way—even as a witness—has serious and long-lasting negative consequences for youth.

- Youth who reported witnessing bullying had greater feelings of helplessness and less sense of connectedness to school than youth who did not report witnessing bullying.

Looking Ahead

There is a lot of concern, even panic, about the ongoing problem of bullying and suicide-related behavior among school-age youth. Much of the media coverage is focused on blame and criminal justice intervention rather than evidence-based, action-oriented prevention. Public health researchers are continually seeking a better understanding of the relationship between bullying and suicide-related behavior as well as the related risk and protective factors that affect young people.

Part Three
Recognizing And Treating Suicidal Ideation

Chapter 23
Why Does A Person Consider Suicide?

Feeling Suicidal

It's a sad truth that teens sometimes think about ending their lives. If you are feeling awful, you may think that suicide is the only answer—but it's not! Don't let suicide be the ending of your story. People want to help, and you can feel better.

It is important to note that suicide is not a normal response to stress. Suicidal thoughts or actions are a sign of extreme distress, not a harmless bid for attention, and should not be ignored.

If You Know Someone In Crisis

Call the toll-free National Suicide Prevention Lifeline at 800-273-TALK (800-273-8255), 24 hours a day, 7 days a week. The service is available to everyone. The deaf and hard of hearing can contact the Lifeline via TTY at 800-799-4889. All calls are confidential.

(Source: "Suicide Prevention," National Institute of Mental Health (NIMH).)

Why Do Some Teens Think About Suicide?

Some teens feel so terrible and overwhelmed that they think life will never get better. Some things that may cause these feelings include:

- the death of someone close

About This Chapter: This chapter includes text excerpted from "Feeling Suicidal," girlshealth.gov, Office on Women's Health (OWH), January 7, 2015.

- having depression or other mental health issues, such as an eating disorder, attention deficit hyperactivity disorder (ADHD), or anxiety

- having alcohol or drug problems

- parents getting divorced

- seeing a lot of anger and violence at home

- having a hard time in school

- being bullied

- having problems with friends

- experiencing a trauma like being raped or abused

- being angry or heartbroken over a relationship break-up

- feeling like you don't belong, either in your family or with friends

- feeling rejected because of something about you, like being gay

- having an ongoing illness or disability

- feeling alone

- feeling guilty or like a burden to other people

Also, teens sometimes may feel very bad for no one clear reason.

If you are suffering, know that things definitely can get better. You can learn ways to handle your feelings. You can work toward a much brighter future.

Turning to others can help you through tough times. If you don't feel a strong connection to relatives or friends, try talking to a school counselor, teacher, doctor, or another adult you trust.

Every teen feels anxiety, sadness, and confusion at some point. The important thing to remember is that life can get much better. There is always help out there for you or a friend.

How Can I Help A Friend Who Has Suicidal Thoughts?

If you think a friend is in immediate danger from suicide call 911 and do not leave him or her alone.

If you think a friend is considering suicide but you're not sure, you can look for some signs. These include:

- talking about not wanting to live

- talking about looking for ways to die, like trying to get pills or a gun
- talking about feeling hopeless or having no purpose
- talking about feeling trapped or being in horrible pain
- talking about being a burden to others
- abusing drugs or alcohol
- acting very nervous or on edge
- doing dangerous things
- sleeping a lot more than before or very little
- not wanting to be around other people
- changing quickly from one strong mood to another
- doing some type of self-injury, like cutting
- acting full of rage or talking about getting revenge
- giving away favorite things

If a friend seems suicidal, ask the person to talk to you about what's going on. Listening shows you care. Remember, though, that you cannot help the person on your own. Encourage your friend to contact a suicide hotline. Suggest that your friend talk to an adult, and possibly offer to go with him or her.

Even if your friend does not want to talk with an adult, you need to tell one as quickly as possible. This can be a relative, school nurse, counselor, teacher, or coach, for example. If you are worried that your friend will be mad, remember that you are doing the right thing. You could save your friend's life.

If a friend posts suicidal thoughts online, you can report the post and help the person get support.

What If I'm Thinking About Suicide?

If you are thinking about suicide, get help right away. You can contact the Lifeline helpline by chat, or call **800-273-TALK (800-273-8255)**. The people there can talk with you about your problems and help you make a plan to stay safe. They also can give you information about ways to get help in person.

If you are in immediate danger of hurting yourself, call 911. You also can go to the nearest hospital emergency department.

Right now, your pain may feel too overwhelming to handle. Suicide may feel like the only way to get relief when you're suffering. But people get past suicidal thoughts, and things can get better.

You can find ways to feel better. Writing is one way to lower your pain. You might list things that you love or your hopes for the future. You also can hang up photos, messages, and other things that remind you that life is worth living. Also, reach out to people who care about you.

Don't try using drugs or alcohol to feel better. These things will not solve your problems. They will only create more problems.

What If Someone I Know Attempts Or Dies By Suicide?

If someone you know attempts or dies by suicide, you may feel like it's your fault in some way. That's not true! You also may feel many different emotions, including anger, grief, or even emotional numbness. All of your feelings are okay. There is not a right or wrong way to feel.

If you are having trouble dealing with your feelings, talk to a trusted adult. You have suffered a terrible loss, but life can feel okay again. Reach out to people who care about you. Connecting is so important at this tough time.

It may be helpful to save several emergency numbers to your cell phone. The ability to get immediate help for yourself or for a friend can make a difference.

- The phone number for a trusted friend or relative.
- The non-emergency number for the local police department.
- The Crisis Text Line: 741741.
- The National Suicide Prevention Lifeline: 800-273-TALK (800-273-8255).

Chapter 24
Types Of Suicidal Thoughts And Behaviors

Suicidal Thoughts

Suicidal ideation: Suicidal ideation is much more common than suicidal behavior. Suicidal ideation lies on a continuum of severity from fleeting and vague thoughts of death to those that are persistent and highly specific. Serious suicidal ideation is frequent, intense, and perceived as uncontrollable.

Suicide plans: Suicide plans are important because they signal more serious risk to carry out suicidal behavior than suicidal ideation that does not involve planning. Suicide planning lies on a continuum from vague and unrealistic plans to those that are highly specific and feasible. Serious suicide planning may also involve rehearsal or preparation for a suicide attempt.

Suicidal Behaviors

Suicide attempt: A suicide attempt is a deliberate act of self-harm that does not result in death and that has at least some intent to die. Attempts have two major elements:

- the subjective level of intent to die (from the client's subjective perspective, how intensely did he or she want to die and to what extent did he or she expect to die?); and

- the objective lethality of the act (from a medical perspective, how likely was it that the behavior would have led to death?)

Although all suicide attempts are serious, those with high intent (the person clearly wanted to die and expected to die) and high lethality (behavior could have easily led to death) are the most serious.

About This Chapter: This chapter includes text excerpted from "Addressing Suicidal Thoughts And Behaviors In Substance Abuse Treatment," Substance Abuse and Mental Health Services Administration (SAMHSA), 2015.

Suicide: Suicide is an acute, deliberate act of self-harm with at least some intention to die resulting in death.

Other Suicide-Related Concepts

Suicidal intention: Suicidal intention (also called "intent") signals high, acute risk for suicidal behavior. Having suicidal intent is always serious because it signals that the client "intends" to make a suicide attempt. Some indicators of "high intent" include drafting a suicide note or taking precautions against discovery at the time of an attempt.

Suicide preparation: Behaviors that suggest preparation signal high, acute risk for suicidal behavior. Preparation may come in many forms, such as writing a suicide note or diary entry, giving away possessions, writing a will, acquiring a method of suicide (e.g., hoarding pills, buying a weapon), making a method more available (e.g., moving a gun from the attic to beside the bed), visiting a site where suicide may be carried out (e.g., driving to a bridge), rehearsing suicide (e.g., loading and unloading a weapon), and saying goodbye to loved ones directly or symbolically.

Other Harmful Behaviors

Non-suicidal self-injury (NSSI): NSSI is also commonly referred to in the literature as "deliberate self-harm" and "suicidal gesture." NSSI (for example, self-mutilation or self-injury by cutting for the purpose of self-soothing with no wish to die and no expectation of dying) is distinguished from a suicide attempt or suicide because NSSI does not include suicidal intent. Suicidal behaviors and NSSI can co-exist in the same person and both can lead to serious bodily injury.

Self-destructive behaviors: Behaviors that are repeated and may eventually lead to death (e.g., drug abuse, smoking, anorexia, pattern of reckless driving, getting into fights) are distinguished from suicidal behavior because an act of suicide is an acute action intended to bring on death in the short term.

Suicide Versus Suicide Attempt

Prevalence: Suicide attempts are much more common than suicides. In the United States, there are approximately 32,000 suicides annually (National Center for Injury Prevention and Control (NCIPC)). More than 10 times that number of self-inflicted injuries were reported in 2006, although the proportion of these injuries in which there was intent to die is unknown (NCIPC).

Suicide Methods: The most common method of attempted suicide is an attempt to overdose. Cutting (for instance, wrists) with a knife is also common.

Lethality: Use of a firearm and hanging are the most lethal methods of suicide. The most common method of death by suicide is firearms, followed by hanging (NCIPC). Attempts by overdose and self-cutting are much more likely to be survived.

Chapter 25

Understanding The Risk, Protective Factors, And Warning Signs Of Suicide

Suicide is the third leading cause of death among persons aged 10–14, the second among persons aged 15–34 years, the fourth among persons aged 35–44 years, the fifth among persons aged 45–54 years, the eighth among person 55–64 years, and the seventeenth among persons 65 years and older.

(Source: "Suicide: At A Glance," National Center for Injury Prevention and Control, Centers for Disease Control and Prevention (CDC).)

Risk Factors For Suicide

A combination of individual, relationship, community, and societal factors contribute to the risk of suicide. Risk factors are those characteristics associated with suicide—they might not be direct causes.

Risk Factors:

- Family history of suicide

- Family history of child maltreatment

- Previous suicide attempt(s)

About This Chapter: Text beginning with the heading "Risk Factors For Suicide" is excerpted from "Suicide: Risk And Protective Factors," Centers for Disease Control and Prevention (CDC), August 15, 2016; Text under the heading "Warning Signs Of Suicidal Behavior" is excerpted from "Suicide Prevention," Substance Abuse and Mental Health Services Administration (SAMHSA), October 29, 2015.

- History of mental disorders, particularly clinical depression

- History of alcohol and substance abuse

- Feelings of hopelessness

- Impulsive or aggressive tendencies

- Cultural and religious beliefs (e.g., belief that suicide is noble resolution of a personal dilemma)

- Local epidemics of suicide

- Isolation, a feeling of being cut off from other people

- Barriers to accessing mental health treatment

- Loss (relational, social, work, or financial)

- Physical illness

- Easy access to lethal methods

- Unwillingness to seek help because of the stigma attached to mental health and substance abuse disorders or to suicidal thoughts

Protective Factors For Suicide

Protective factors buffer individuals from suicidal thoughts and behavior. To date, protective factors have not been studied as extensively or rigorously as risk factors. Identifying and understanding protective factors are, however, equally as important as researching risk factors.

Protective Factors:

- Effective clinical care for mental, physical, and substance abuse disorders

- Easy access to a variety of clinical interventions and support for help-seeking

- Family and community support (connectedness)

- Support from ongoing medical and mental healthcare relationships

- Skills in problem-solving, conflict resolution, and nonviolent ways of handling disputes

- Cultural and religious beliefs that discourage suicide and support instincts for self-preservation

Warning Signs Of Suicidal Behavior

These signs may mean that someone is at risk for suicide. Risk is greater if the behavior is new, or has increased, and if it seems related to a painful event, loss, or change:

- Talking about wanting to die or kill oneself
- Looking for a way to kill oneself
- Talking about feeling hopeless or having no reason to live
- Talking about feeling trapped or being in unbearable pain
- Talking about being a burden to others
- Increasing the use of alcohol or drugs
- Acting anxious or agitated; behaving recklessly
- Sleeping too little or too much
- Withdrawing or feeling isolated
- Showing rage or talking about seeking revenge
- Displaying extreme mood swings

What You Can Do

If you believe someone may be thinking about suicide:

- Ask them if they are thinking about killing themselves. (This will not put the idea into their head or make it more likely that they will attempt suicide.)
- Listen without judging and show you care.
- Stay with the person (or make sure the person is in a private, secure place with another caring person) until you can get further help.
- Remove any objects that could be used in a suicide attempt.
- Call SAMHSA's National Suicide Prevention Lifeline at 800-273-TALK (800-273-8255) and follow their guidance.
- If danger for self-harm seems imminent, call 911.

Everyone has a role to play in preventing suicide. For instance, faith communities can work to prevent suicide simply by fostering cultures and norms that are life-preserving, providing perspective and social support to community members, and helping people navigate the struggles of life to find a sustainable sense of hope, meaning, and purpose.

Chapter 26
Recovering From A Suicide Attempt

How Did It Get To This Point?

The time right after your suicide attempt can be the most confusing and emotional part of your entire life. In some ways, it may be even more difficult than the time preceding your attempt. Not only are you still facing the thoughts and feelings that led you to consider suicide, but now you may be struggling to figure out what to do since you survived.

It's likely that your decision to try to kill yourself didn't come out of the blue. It probably developed over time, perhaps from overwhelming feelings that seemed too much to bear. Experiencing these emotions might have been especially difficult if you had to deal with them alone. A variety of stressful situations can lead to suicidal feelings, including the loss of a loved one, relationship issues, financial difficulties, health problems, trauma, depression, or other mental health concerns. It's possible that you were experiencing some of these problems when you started to think about suicide.

While the events that lead to a suicide attempt can vary from person to person, a common theme that many suicide attempt survivors report is the need to feel relief. At desperate moments, when it feels like nothing else is working, suicide may seem like the only way to get relief from unbearable emotional pain.

Just as it took time for the pain that led to your suicide attempt to become unbearable, it may also take some time for it to subside. That's okay. The important thing is that you're still here; you're alive, which means you have time to find healthier and more effective ways to cope with your pain.

About This Chapter: This chapter includes text excerpted from "A Journey Toward Health And Hope," Substance Abuse and Mental Health Services Administration (SAMHSA), 2015.

What Am I Feeling Right Now?

Right now, you're probably experiencing many conflicting emotions.

You may be thinking:

- "Why am I still here? I wish I were dead. I couldn't even do this right."

- "I don't know if I can get through this. I don't even have the energy to try."

- "I can't do this alone."

- "How do I tell anyone about this? What do I say to them? What will they think of me?"

- "Maybe someone will pay attention to me now; maybe someone will help me."

- "Maybe there is a reason I survived. How do I figure out what that reason is?"

Right after a suicide attempt, many survivors have said that the pain that led them to harm themselves as still present. Some felt angry that they survived their attempt. Others felt embarrassed, ashamed, or guilty that they put their family and friends through a difficult situation. Most felt alone and said they had no idea how to go on living. They didn't know what to expect and even questioned whether they had the strength to stay alive. Still others felt that if they survived their attempt, there must be some reason they were still alive, and they wanted to discover why.

You're probably experiencing some of the same feelings and may be wondering how others have faced these challenges. Some examples of the steps others found helpful in recovering from a suicide attempt is provided below.

Am I the Only One Who Feels This Way?

Knowing how others made it through can help you learn new ways to recover from your own suicide attempt.

It's estimated that more than one million people attempt suicide each year in the United States, from all parts of society. In other words, you're not alone. However, it can be hard to know how other survivors recovered because suicide is a personal topic that often is not discussed openly and honestly. This can leave those affected feeling like they don't know where to turn.

Shame, dreading the reaction of others, or fear of being hospitalized are some of the reasons that prevent people from talking about suicide. This is unfortunate, because direct and open communication about suicide can help prevent people from acting on suicidal thoughts. Hopefully, reading about the experiences of other survivors will make it easier for you to talk about your own attempt, learn ways to keep yourself safe, know when to ask for help, and most importantly, find hope as you think about what happens next on your journey.

It's okay if you feel conflicting emotions right now. Other suicide attempt survivors know that what you're experiencing is normal. They understand that your concerns are real. Going on won't be easy, and finding a way to ease your emotional pain may be challenging, but this can be a time to start down a new path toward a better life—to start your journey toward help and hope.

Taking The First Steps

Recovery is a process, and it's important that you move at your own pace. There are a few things you might want to do to ease your transition back to everyday life. Some important steps that others have found helpful are listed below.

Talking With Others About Your Attempt

One of the most difficult tasks you might face will be responding to the questions people ask about your suicide attempt. The shame, guilt, confusion, and other emotions that might follow an attempt can make it tough to speak about it with others, especially if people respond in a way that doesn't feel supportive.

Often, those closest to you may be feeling lots of emotions about your attempt. They may be scared, confused, or angry about what happened, causing them to focus on their own feelings, rather than being as supportive as you need them to be. Their reactions might hurt you, whether they mean to or not.

To make it easier, here are some suggestions that can be helpful:

It's your story to tell, or not.

The details of your experience are personal, and it's up to you to determine what you want to share and with whom. Sharing what happened with your doctors, nurses, counselor, or peer supporters can help them give you the right kind of support. In most cases, they're required to keep the details of what you share confidential.

You may want to share some of the details and your feelings about what happened with other people you trust, such as family or friends. How much you share, or the details you decide to give, are up to you and what you feel comfortable with.

People don't always say the right things.

It's difficult to predict how people will respond when they learn that you tried to kill yourself. Some people might change the subject or avoid the topic altogether because of their fear of death or suicide. Others who are close to you may be confused, hurt, or angry about what's happened. They may judge or blame you. They may feel betrayed or be wondering what they could have done to prevent you from attempting suicide.

Often, those who care the most about you have the strongest reactions to your suicide attempt because they can't imagine life without you. It's helpful to remember that a strong reaction may reflect your family's or friends' depth of concern about you.

Sometimes you may feel that they're being overly controlling. It may seem like they're watching everything you do or won't leave you alone because they're afraid you may attempt suicide again. This can be very frustrating when you're trying to recover from an attempt.

It can take time to repair the trust in your relationships. If you can show that you're committed to safety, it might allow those close to you to feel more comfortable giving you the space you need. Completing a safety plan, can help you show those who are worried about you that you want to stay safe.

Direct communication may help you get what you need.

While it may be hard for you to talk about what happened, it is also important for you to try your best to be direct in communicating what you need. It may seem obvious to you, but others may not understand or know the best way to support you. This period can be challenging because you might want to ask people for help, but you don't want to scare anyone if you're still struggling. This is especially true if you're concerned that people might overreact and insist on care in a hospital when you believe you just need more support and understanding.

Support can make things easier.

It might be hard at first, but having someone you feel comfortable talking to after your attempt is very important. You may face some challenges as you move forward; knowing there is at least one person you can turn to will make the road to recovery less daunting. Being alone with suicidal thoughts can be dangerous. Having supportive people around you and educating them on how to help you can be a crucial part of staying safe.

Ask yourself, "What do I need from a support person?"

Different people need different things after a suicide attempt, so make sure the person you choose meets your unique needs. Maybe you need someone who will listen to you without judgment, or maybe you need someone who will come and be with you when you're feeling alone. Perhaps it would be helpful to have someone close to you who can go with you to appointments, or perhaps you want to schedule regular phone calls with a trusted friend. No matter what kind of assistance you need, it's helpful to have at least one person with whom you can share your thoughts of suicide—someone who will stay calm and help you when you need support. And remember, because you might not get everything you need from one person, it can be helpful to have a variety of people available to support you, if possible.

Re-Establishing Connections

It's likely that the overwhelming life events, stress, and depression that led to your suicide attempt affected your ability to enjoy life. Struggling with suicidal thoughts can be exhausting and leave you with little energy to do the things you once loved. It also can put stress on your relationships with friends and family. The irony of depression and suicidal thinking is that they may cause you to give up the things in life that help you feel better, just when you need them the most.

> Even up until the moment of their attempts, many suicide attempt survivors report that there was an internal struggle going on inside them. One side argued that suicide was the best way to end the pain they were experiencing. The other side struggled to find another way to feel better. To put it another way, most people with suicidal thoughts had reasons for dying AND reasons for living.

Before your suicide attempt, you might have lost connections to your reasons for living, but it's important to re-establish those connections because they can help instill hope. They can remind you about the things you love in life.

Planning To Stay Safe

You might still have thoughts of suicide after your attempt, even if you've decided that you want to stay alive. Perhaps the pain that led to your suicide attempt is still there. It's okay to have suicidal thoughts. Everyone needs to feel relief from unbearable pain, and suicidal thoughts may be one of the ways you've learned to cope. What's important is that you don't act on those thoughts and that you try to find other, safer ways to ease your pain. A safety plan can help you do this.

What Is A Safety Plan?

A safety plan is a written list of coping strategies and resources to help you survive a suicidal crisis. A safety plan can help you discover other ways to ease your pain so you don't feel tempted to act on suicidal thoughts you may experience.

Your plan will be a personalized list of strategies to help you cope. You can use these strategies before or during a suicidal crisis. By writing them down, you'll always know what they are, even if you're upset or not thinking clearly.

You can complete your plan by yourself or with the help of a counselor, peer, family member, or friend. The following questions will help you brainstorm elements of your safety plan.

1. **What triggers my suicidal thoughts?**

   Many suicide attempt survivors indicate that their suicidal thinking became almost automatic over time. When something negative occurred, they would start to have negative thoughts.

   It may have been an event or behavior (called triggers), such as failing a test, not sleeping well, or arguing with a loved one, that led to suicidal thoughts. Some survivors noticed that their suicidal thoughts occurred with a certain mood, such as feeling angry or sad, while others started feeling suicidal when remembering a painful event from the past. No matter what the trigger, many survivors experienced a common theme: When something negative occurred, they would start thinking things like:

   • "I'm no good." "I can't do anything right." "I fail at everything I do."

   • "I hate myself. I'm worthless." "I don't want to be here anymore."

   • "Nobody cares about me."

   • "I can't take it anymore. I wish I were dead."

   Coping with these types of negative thoughts can be difficult. If you don't talk about how you're feeling with someone, the thoughts might start to escalate. One survivor indicated that it was like having "tunnel vision." Even though her negative thoughts weren't always true, the feelings they created became so strong that she started to believe them.

   It's important to recognize what triggers your suicidal thoughts for several reasons, but the most important reason is to recognize when you're in crisis and that it's time to use your safety plan.

2. **What can I do to take my mind off these thoughts?**

   While suicidal thoughts after an attempt may be common, it's important to find ways to keep them from escalating into suicidal behaviors. One way is to do something that helps you feel better and takes your mind off your problems. For this step of the safety plan, you should think of internal coping strategies or things you can do when you're by yourself. These strategies vary from person to person.

3. **Where can I go or with whom can I talk to feel better?**

Another way to take your mind off your suicidal thoughts is through external strategies, like talking to certain people or visiting places that improve your mood. Finding places that make you feel better or people who cheer you up are good ways to keep your thoughts from escalating.

4. **Whom can I ask for help? Who knows that I'm struggling with thoughts of suicide?**

If the ideas above don't seem to be helping, you may need more specific assistance, like talking to someone with whom you feel comfortable sharing your thoughts of suicide. Ideally, this is a support person who already knows about your suicidal thoughts and is aware of his or her role as a support person in your plan. If it's difficult for you to ask people for support, you might say, "I'm calling you today because I feel like I might need to use my safety plan."

5. **What resources can I contact if I'm in crisis?**

The next step of the plan involves contacting professionals who can offer assistance if the other parts of the plan don't seem to be increasing your ability to stay safe. Ideally, you want to have resources that are available 24 hours a day, 7 days a week. The National Suicide Prevention Lifeline 800-273-TALK (800-273-8255) is a resource that's always available.

6. **Are there items around me that may put me in danger?**

While suicide may seem like a quick way to end your pain, it can have devastating consequences for you and the people who care about you. You can use your safety plan to help find alternate ways of relieving your pain that don't involve ending your life. However, if you forget to use your plan, or it doesn't make you feel better, having items close to you that you could use to harm yourself can create a dangerous situation. It's important, then, to remove items that you may use impulsively in a moment of unbearable pain.

Most suicide attempt survivors indicate that their thoughts of suicide changed over time. While they had periods when the pain seemed unbearable, those times didn't last forever. Removing dangerous items gives you time to allow the way you're feeling to change.

7. **Incorporating reasons for living and hope into your safety plan**

    Depression and suicidal thinking tend to make you focus only on your reasons for dying, while not allowing you to appreciate your reasons for living. It can be helpful to add your reasons for living into your safety plan as reminders of the things in life that are important to you, as well as the people whom you care about and who care about you. Reminding yourself of your reasons for living can help build hope and increase your motivation to stay safe.

What Should You Do With Your Plan?

Your plan is for your use, but it's a good idea to share it with a few other people. Your support person and backup person can do a better job in times of crisis if they have your most recent copy. If you're using a paper safety plan, you may want to keep multiple copies in various places so it's nearby whenever you need it. Your safety plan may change over time. You can add information to it in the future as you identify more triggers or want to change the names of contacts. You wouldn't want to search around for information in a crisis situation, so it's a good idea to keep contact information up-to-date.

There's one more thing about your safety plan that's very important—you have to actually use it! It's important to think about ways you can use it when you're afraid your suicidal thoughts might escalate to suicidal actions. For this reason, it should contain items and ideas that work for you, not things you feel others are forcing you to do. If you don't like the options or you feel they're unrealistic, say so. If you can't find options that are right for you, this may indicate that you need more support until you feel comfortable that you can stay safe.

Finding A Counselor

Suicide attempt survivors and researchers who study suicide recommend professional help as your best bet for finding long-term strategies to ease the emotional pain that led to your attempt.

Making a decision to go to therapy can be intimidating. You might worry that it will be uncomfortable or that it could lead to hospitalization, but most people who give it a try find it really helps.

When looking for a counselor, it might be difficult to know where to start. It's always smart to ask others which counselors in your area have good reputations. Your doctor or the people that helped you in the emergency room might have suggestions. Here are other ideas:

- Call the National Suicide Prevention Lifeline 800-273-TALK (800-273-8255). Lifeline crisis workers know their local communities and may be able to refer you to a counselor or support group in your area.

- Check out the SAMHSA Behavioral Health Treatment Services Locator online at findtreatment.samhsa.gov or call them at 800-662-HELP (800-662-4357).

- In many communities, you can reach an information and referral hotline by dialing three simple digits: 2-1-1. If dialing 2-1-1 doesn't work for you, check out www.211.org for the seven-digit number of your local information and referral hotline.

- Try the Suicide Prevention Therapist Finder: www.helppro.com/SPTF/BasicSearch.aspx

- You can also check with a local chapter of a mental health organization, such as the American Psychiatric Association, American Psychological Association, Anxiety Disorders Association of America (ADAA), Mental Health America (MHA), National Alliance on Mental Illness (NAMI), or Depression and Bipolar Support Alliance (DBSA).

Chapter 27
Going To A Therapist: What To Expect

Lots of teens have some kind of emotional problem. In fact, almost half of U.S. teens will have a mental health problem before they turn 18. The good news is that therapy can really help.

Sometimes, people are embarrassed or afraid to see a therapist. But getting help from a therapist because you're feeling sad or anxious is really not different from seeing a doctor because you broke a bone. In fact, you can feel proud for being brave enough to do what you need to do to get your life back on track.

Here are some common questions and answers about therapy.

What Is Therapy?

Therapy is when you talk about your problems with someone who is a professional counselor, such as a psychiatrist, psychologist, or social worker. Therapy sometimes is called psychotherapy. That is because it helps with your psychology—the mental and emotional parts of your life.

If you are going through a rough time, talking to a caring therapist can be a great relief. A therapist can help you cope with sadness, worry, and other strong or scary feelings. Here are some other ways therapy can help:

- It can teach you specific skills for handling difficult situations, such as problems with your family or school.
- It can help you find healthy ways to deal with stress or anger.
- It can teach you how to build healthy relationships.
- It can help you figure out how to think about things in more positive ways.

About This Chapter: This chapter includes text excerpted from "Going To Therapy," girlshealth.gov, Office on Women's Health (OWH), January 7, 2015.

- It can help you figure out how to boost your self-confidence.
- It can help you decide where you want to go in life and how to deal with any obstacles that may come up along the way.

Therapy may feel great right away, or it might feel strange at first. It can take a little time getting used to talking with someone new about your problems. But therapists are trained to listen well, and they want to help.

As time goes on, you should feel comfortable with your therapist. If you don't feel comfortable, or if you think you're not getting better, tell your parent or guardian. Another therapist or type of therapy might work better.

Therapists protect people's privacy. They can share what you say only in very special cases, such as if they think you are in danger. If you're concerned, though, ask about the privacy policy. It's important to feel like you can tell the truth in therapy. It works best if you are honest about any problems you're facing, including problems with drugs or alcohol or any behaviors that can hurt your body or mind.

Just because you start to see a therapist doesn't mean that you will see one forever. You should be able to learn skills that let you handle your problems on your own. Sometimes, a few sessions are all you need to learn skills and feel better.

Why Do Teens Go For Therapy?

Many young people develop mental health conditions, like depression, eating disorders, or anxiety disorders. If you have a mental health problem, remember there are treatments that work, and you can feel better. Also, some teens go to therapy to get help through a tough time, like their parents' getting divorced or having too much stress at school.

If you feel out of control, or you feel like a mental health problem keeps you from enjoying life, get help. Reach out to a parent or guardian or another trusted adult.

What Should I Do To Get Started With Therapy?

If you need help finding a therapist, you can start by talking to your doctor, school nurse, or school counselor. If your family has insurance, the insurance company can tell you which therapists are covered under your plan. You and your parent or guardian also can look online for mental health treatment.

If you need help paying for therapy, you can ask a parent or guardian if they have health insurance that might help pay for therapy. If your family doesn't have insurance, they can find out about getting it through the website, www.healthcare.gov. You also may be able to get free or low-cost therapy at a mental health clinic, hospital, university, or other places.

What Are Some Kinds Of Therapy?

There are different kinds of therapy to help you feel better. The best treatment depends on the type of problem that you are facing.

You may have one-on-one talk therapy. This is when you talk to a therapist alone. Or you may join group therapy, where you work with a therapist and other people who are having similar issues. You may also do art therapy, where you paint or draw.

One kind of talk therapy that tends to work well for depression, anxiety, and several other problems is cognitive behavioral therapy. This type of therapy teaches you how to think and act in healthier ways.

Sometimes, your therapist will suggest that you take medicine in addition to therapy, which often can be a helpful combination.

What Is Talk Therapy?

Talk therapy is a type of treatment in which you talk with a trained therapist. You may meet with the therapist one-on-one or in a group. Sessions are usually once a week. If you try talk therapy, you should have at least eight sessions to see if it helps.

Talking with a therapist about issues that have to do with your depression may upset you. You may feel angry, nervous, or sad. Working through these feelings may be part of getting better. It is important to tell your therapist if talk therapy upsets you or if your depression symptoms get worse.

Types Of Talk Therapy And How It Helps

- **Cognitive behavioral therapy:** You learn to notice your negative thoughts and actions so you can replace them with positive ones.
- **Interpersonal therapy:** You work on problems you have with people in your life and learn new ways to communicate.
- **Psychodynamic therapy:** You uncover deep feelings and past experiences to learn how they affect the way you feel and act now.

Researchers found that as the first treatment for depression:

- Cognitive behavioral therapy improves depression symptoms as well as antidepressants. People are able to stick with cognitive behavioral therapy as well as they are able to stick with antidepressants.

> • Interpersonal therapy and psychodynamic therapy may improve depression symptoms about as well as antidepressants, but more research is needed to know for sure. Only a few studies have been done on these types of talk therapy.
>
> *(Source: "Comparing Talk Therapy And Other Depression Treatments With Antidepressant Medicines," Agency for Healthcare Research and Quality (AHRQ), U.S. Department of Health and Human Services (HHS).)*

What About Online Support Groups?

There are lots of support groups available on the Internet, including ones to help you handle your feelings. Chat rooms and other online options may help you feel less alone. But if you are having trouble coping, it's important to work with a therapist or other mental health professional.

Remember to be careful about getting information online. Some people use the Internet to promote unhealthy behaviors, like cutting and dangerous eating habits. Learn to be safe on the Internet.

eHealth

The telephone, Internet, and mobile devices have opened up new possibilities for providing interventions that can reach people in areas where mental health professionals may be not be easily available, and can be at hand 24/7. Some of these approaches involve a therapist providing help at a distance, but others—such as web-based programs and cell phone apps—are designed to provide information and feedback in the absence of a therapist.

Chapter 28
Getting What You Need From Counseling

Selecting a counselor is an important decision, and you'll find many options for various types of therapy. When choosing a counselor, it's vital to find someone who is comfortable with and has experience talking about suicide. It's also important to remember that if drugs or alcohol played a part in the problems that led to your suicide attempt, your counselor should have experience in substance abuse treatment.

Medication could be an important part of your path to recovery, especially if you've ever been diagnosed with major depression, bipolar disorder, schizophrenia, or an anxiety disorder, or if your symptoms are so troubling that you're having problems getting through the day. This might include having serious problems sleeping; having no appetite or eating too much; thinking negative thoughts that you can't stop, no matter how hard you try; or hearing voices. If this sounds like you, you'll want to discuss medication with your counselor. Together you can find a doctor or psychiatrist who can work with you to determine whether medication might be helpful.

Different people have different needs, and sometimes it takes time to find a counselor who is right for you. This can be a frustrating process, but if one counselor, doctor, or type of therapy doesn't work, you have the right to keep trying until you find one that does. Think about your preferences in a counselor (or clinician, therapist, doctor, or psychiatrist): a man or a woman, their age range, ethinicity, language, etc. If you have a choice of counselors, call ahead for an interview or use the first session to get to know them better. Ask questions to see if they might be a good match for your style and needs. Remember, it's crucial that you be persistent. Any

About This Chapter: This chapter includes text excerpted from "A Journey Toward Health And Hope," Substance Abuse and Mental Health Services Administration (SAMHSA), 2015.

important decision requires some research, and sometimes it takes trial and error before you get it right.

While there are many different approaches to therapy, research shows that the following methods are especially helpful for those struggling with suicidal thoughts and attempts:

- Cognitive behavioral therapy (CBT)

- Dialectical behavior therapy (DBT)

- Collaborative Assessment and Management of Suicidality (CAMS)

The Lifeline was mentioned earlier as a source for finding referrals for counselors, but it's also a great place for support if you're in crisis. While not a substitute for ongoing therapy, the Lifeline is a network of confidential crisis hotlines across the country that are staffed by trained crisis workers. This means they won't be shocked or scared by what you say, and, importantly, they won't judge you. Lifeline crisis workers will talk with you about your suicidal feelings and brainstorm ways to help you stay safe. Crisis workers are available 24 hours a day, 7 days a week. Best of all, it's a free service.

If You Don't Go To Counseling

While it might be easier to recover from your suicide attempt with the help of a counselor, you may choose to try to get better on your own. This might be because you don't have insurance and can't afford counseling. Maybe you tried counseling, but had difficulty finding a counselor who was right for you. Maybe you don't feel like taking that step right now. It's important to remember that if struggles with a mental illness led to your suicide attempt, it might be difficult to get better and recover on your own. Just as with some physical ailments, you may find it particularly challenging to heal without medications or help from a professional.

Whatever your reason for not seeing a counselor, there are things you can do to get better on your own. The ideas already mentioned here are a good start. When you're ready, you might find the following options to be helpful as well. And even if you do have a counselor, these ideas can be great resources for additional support.

Call the National Suicide Prevention Lifeline.

The Lifeline can be a great resource for your friends and family as well. If they're having difficulty understanding your struggles with suicide or don't know how to support you, a crisis worker can speak to them about their concerns and give them ideas on how to help. Evaluations of crisis hotlines have shown that they can reduce emotional distress and suicidal thinking in callers.

If talking about suicide is difficult for you, you may want to check out the Lifeline website, www.suicidepreventionlifeline.org.

Join a support group.

A support group is composed of people who meet regularly to talk about common concerns and look out for each other's well-being. Support groups can be helpful because they allow you to meet others who have had experiences similar to yours. It can be a huge relief to learn that you're not alone and that there are others who feel the way you do. It also can be helpful to learn about strategies others have found useful.

Just as there are different types of counselors, there are support groups for a variety of topics, such as:

- depression
- anxiety
- substance abuse
- self-esteem
- anger
- posttraumatic stress, sexual assault, and other traumas
- hearing voices (e.g., schizophrenia)

A few communities across the country are even beginning to offer support groups **specifically for people who have survived a suicide attempt** or who are struggling with persistent thoughts of suicide.

Many times, support groups are led by an experienced counselor; other times they are peer-led by people who have experienced similar issues. If you don't have insurance to pay for individual counseling, a group may be one way to get help. They are often free of charge or much less expensive than seeing an individual counselor.

The information and referral hotline in your community (dial 2-1-1 or visit www.211. org) or the Lifeline 800-273-TALK (800-273-8255) or www.suicidepreventionlifeline.org) can give you more information about support groups in your area.

Read books or visit websites.

Sometimes, if you aren't ready or don't have access to a counselor, you can find helpful information on your own. There are many websites and books that address issues related to stress, depression, or other mental health issues. There are even several books written by people who have survived a suicide attempt.

Chapter 29

Medications For Treatment Of Mental Health Disorders

Medications

Medications can play a role in treating several mental disorders and conditions. Treatment may also include psychotherapy (also called "talk therapy") and brain stimulation therapies (less common). In some cases, psychotherapy alone may be the best treatment option. Choosing the right treatment plan should be based on a person's individual needs and medical situation, and under a mental health professional's care.

Many medications used to treat children and adolescents with mental illness are safe and effective. However, some medications have not been studied or approved for use with children or adolescents.

Still, a doctor can give a young person an FDA-approved medication on an "off-label" basis. This means that the doctor prescribes the medication to help the patient even though the medicine is not approved for the specific mental disorder that is being treated or for use by patients under a certain age. Remember:

- It is important to watch children and adolescents who take these medications on an "off-label" basis.

- Children may have different reactions and side effects than adults.

- Some medications have current FDA warnings about potentially dangerous side effects for younger patients.

About This Chapter: This chapter includes text excerpted from "Mental Health Medications," National Institute of Mental Health (NIMH), October 2016.

In addition to medications, other treatments for children and adolescents should be considered, either to be tried first, with medication added later if necessary, or to be provided along with medication. Psychotherapy, family therapy, educational courses, and behavior management techniques can help everyone involved cope with disorders that affect a child's mental health.

Understanding Your Medications

If you are prescribed a medication, be sure that you:

- Tell the doctor about all medications and vitamin supplements you are already taking.
- Remind your doctor about any allergies and any problems you have had with medicines.
- Understand how to take the medicine before you start using it and take your medicine as instructed.
- Don't take medicines prescribed for another person or give yours to someone else.
- Call your doctor right away if you have any problems with your medicine or if you are worried that it might be doing more harm than good. Your doctor may be able to adjust the dose or change your prescription to a different one that may work better for you.

Antidepressants

Antidepressants are medications commonly used to treat depression. Antidepressants are also used for other health conditions, such as anxiety, pain and insomnia. Although antidepressants are not U.S. Food and Drug Administration (FDA) approved specifically to treat attention deficit hyperactivity disorder (ADHD), antidepressants are sometimes used to treat ADHD in adults.

The most popular types of antidepressants are called selective serotonin reuptake inhibitors (SSRIs). Examples of SSRIs include:

- Fluoxetine
- Citalopram
- Sertraline
- Paroxetine
- Escitalopram

Other types of antidepressants are serotonin and norepinephrine reuptake inhibitors (SNRIs). SNRIs are similar to SSRIs and include venlafaxine and duloxetine.

Another antidepressant that is commonly used is bupropion. Bupropion is a third type of antidepressant which works differently than either SSRIs or SNRIs. Bupropion is also used to treat seasonal affective disorder and to help people stop smoking.

SSRIs, SNRIs, and bupropion are popular because they do not cause as many side effects as older classes of antidepressants, and seem to help a broader group of depressive and anxiety disorders. Older antidepressant medications include tricyclics, tetracyclics, and monoamine oxidase inhibitors (MAOIs). For some people, tricyclics, tetracyclics, or MAOIs may be the best medications.

How Do People Respond To Antidepressants?

According to a research review by the Agency for Healthcare Research and Quality (AHRQ), all antidepressant medications work about as well as each other to improve symptoms of depression and to keep depression symptoms from coming back. For reasons not yet well understood, some people respond better to some antidepressant medications than to others.

Therefore, it is important to know that some people may not feel better with the first medicine they try and may need to try several medicines to find the one that works for them. Others may find that a medicine helped for a while, but their symptoms came back. It is important to carefully follow your doctor's directions for taking your medicine at an adequate dose and over an extended period of time (often 4 to 6 weeks) for it to work.

Once a person begins taking antidepressants, it is important to not stop taking them without the help of a doctor. Sometimes people taking antidepressants feel better and stop taking the medication too soon, and the depression may return. When it is time to stop the medication, the doctor will help the person slowly and safely decrease the dose. It's important to give the body time to adjust to the change. People don't get addicted (or "hooked") on these medications, but stopping them abruptly may also cause withdrawal symptoms.

What Are The Possible Side Effects Of Antidepressants?

Some antidepressants may cause more side effects than others. You may need to try several different antidepressant medications before finding the one that improves your symptoms and that causes side effects that you can manage.

The most common side effects listed by the FDA include:

- nausea and vomiting
- weight gain

- diarrhea

- sleepiness

- sexual problems

Call your doctor right away if you have any of the following symptoms, especially if they are new, worsening, or worry you:

- thoughts about suicide or dying

- attempts to commit suicide

- new or worsening depression

- new or worsening anxiety

- feeling very agitated or restless

- panic attacks

- trouble sleeping (insomnia)

- new or worsening irritability

- acting aggressively, being angry, or violent

- acting on dangerous impulses

- an extreme increase in activity and talking (mania)

- other unusual changes in behavior or mood

Combining the newer SSRI or SNRI antidepressants with one of the commonly-used "triptan" medications used to treat migraine headaches could cause a life-threatening illness called "serotonin syndrome." A person with serotonin syndrome may be agitated, have hallucinations (see or hear things that are not real), have a high temperature, or have unusual blood pressure changes. Serotonin syndrome is usually associated with the older antidepressants called MAOIs, but it can happen with the newer antidepressants as well, if they are mixed with the wrong medications.

Antidepressants may cause other side effects that were not included in this list.

Anti-Anxiety Medications

What Are Anti-Anxiety Medications?

Anti-anxiety medications help reduce the symptoms of anxiety, such as panic attacks, or extreme fear and worry. The most common anti-anxiety medications are called benzodiazepines.

Benzodiazepines can treat generalized anxiety disorder. In the case of panic disorder or social phobia (social anxiety disorder), benzodiazepines are usually second-line treatments, behind SSRIs or other antidepressants.

Benzodiazepines used to treat anxiety disorders include:

* Clonazepam

* Alprazolam

* Lorazepam

Short half-life (or short-acting) benzodiazepines (such as Lorazepam) and beta blockers are used to treat the short-term symptoms of anxiety. Beta blockers help manage physical symptoms of anxiety, such as trembling, rapid heartbeat, and sweating that people with phobias (an overwhelming and unreasonable fear of an object or situation, such as public speaking) experience in difficult situations. Taking these medications for a short period of time can help the person keep physical symptoms under control and can be used "as needed" to reduce acute anxiety.

Buspirone (which is unrelated to the benzodiazepines) is sometimes used for the long-term treatment of chronic anxiety. In contrast to the benzodiazepines, buspirone must be taken every day for a few weeks to reach its full effect. It is not useful on an "as-needed" basis.

How Do People Respond To Anti-Anxiety Medications?

Anti-anxiety medications such as benzodiazepines are effective in relieving anxiety and take effect more quickly than the antidepressant medications (or buspirone) often prescribed for anxiety. However, people can build up a tolerance to benzodiazepines if they are taken over a long period of time and may need higher and higher doses to get the same effect. Some people may even become dependent on them. To avoid these problems, doctors usually prescribe benzodiazepines for short periods, a practice that is especially helpful for older adults, people who have substance abuse problems and people who become dependent on medication easily. If people suddenly stop taking benzodiazepines, they may have withdrawal symptoms or their anxiety may return. Therefore, benzodiazepines should be tapered off slowly.

What Are The Possible Side Effects Of Anti-Anxiety Medications?

Like other medications, anti-anxiety medications may cause side effects. Some of these side effects and risks are serious. The most common side effects for benzodiazepines are drowsiness and dizziness. Other possible side effects include:

* nausea

- blurred vision

- headache

- confusion

- tiredness

- nightmares

Tell your doctor if any of these symptoms are severe or do not go away:

- drowsiness

- dizziness

- unsteadiness

- problems with coordination

- difficulty thinking or remembering

- increased saliva

- muscle or joint pain

- frequent urination

- blurred vision

- changes in sex drive or ability

If you experience any of the symptoms below, call your doctor immediately:

- rash

- hives

- swelling of the eyes, face, lips, tongue, or throat

- difficulty breathing or swallowing

- hoarseness

- seizures

- yellowing of the skin or eyes

- depression

- difficulty speaking

- thoughts of suicide or harming yourself

Common side effects of beta blockers include:

- fatigue

- cold hands

- dizziness or light-headedness

- weakness

Beta blockers generally are not recommended for people with asthma or diabetes because they may worsen symptoms related to both.

Possible side effects from buspirone include:

- dizziness

- headaches

- nausea

- nervousness

- lightheadedness

- excitement

- trouble sleeping

Anti-anxiety medications may cause other side effects that are not included in the lists above.

Stimulants

As the name suggests, stimulants increase alertness, attention, and energy, as well as elevate blood pressure, heart rate, and respiration. Stimulant medications are often prescribed to treat children, adolescents, or adults diagnosed with ADHD.

Stimulants used to treat ADHD include:

- Methylphenidate

- Amphetamine

- Dextroamphetamine

- Lisdexamfetamine Dimesylate

How Do People Respond To Stimulants?

Prescription stimulants have a calming and "focusing" effect on individuals with ADHD. Stimulant medications are safe when given under a doctor's supervision. Some children taking them may feel slightly different or "funny."

Some parents worry that stimulant medications may lead to drug abuse or dependence, but there is little evidence of this when they are used properly as prescribed. Additionally, research shows that teens with ADHD who took stimulant medications were less likely to abuse drugs than those who did not take stimulant medications.

What Are The Possible Side Effects Of Stimulants?

Stimulants may cause side effects. Most side effects are minor and disappear when dosage levels are lowered. The most common side effects include:

- difficulty falling asleep or staying asleep
- loss of appetite
- stomach pain
- headache

Less common side effects include:

- motor tics or verbal tics (sudden, repetitive movements or sounds)
- personality changes, such as appearing "flat" or without emotion

Call your doctor right away if you have any of these symptoms, especially if they are new, become worse, or worry you.

Stimulants may cause other side effects that are not included in the list above.

Do Prescription Stimulants Make You Smarter?

A growing number of teenagers and young adults are abusing prescription stimulants to boost their study performance in an effort to improve their grades in school, and there is a widespread belief that these drugs can improve a person's ability to learn ("cognitive enhancement").

Prescription stimulants do promote wakefulness, but studies have found that they do not enhance learning or thinking ability when taken by people who do not actually have ADHD. Also, research has shown that students who abuse prescription stimulants actually have lower GPAs in high school and college than those who don't.

(Source: "Stimulant ADHD Medications: Methylphenidate And Amphetamines," National Institute on Drug Abuse (NIDA).)

Antipsychotics

Antipsychotic medicines are primarily used to manage psychosis. The word "psychosis" is used to describe conditions that affect the mind, and in which there has been some loss of contact with reality, often including delusions (false, fixed beliefs) or hallucinations (hearing or seeing things that are not really there). It can be a symptom of a physical condition such as drug abuse or a mental disorder such as schizophrenia, bipolar disorder, or very severe depression (also known as "psychotic depression").

Antipsychotic medications are often used in combination with other medications to treat delirium, dementia, and mental health conditions, including:

- attention deficit hyperactivity disorder (ADHD)

- severe depression

- eating disorders

- posttraumatic stress disorder (PTSD)

- obsessive compulsive disorder (OCD)

- generalized anxiety disorder

Antipsychotic medicines do not cure these conditions. They are used to help relieve symptoms and improve quality of life.

Older or first-generation antipsychotic medications are also called conventional "typical" antipsychotics or "neuroleptics." Some of the common typical antipsychotics include:

- Chlorpromazine

- Haloperidol

- Perphenazine

- Fluphenazine

Newer or second generation medications are also called "atypical" antipsychotics. Some of the common atypical antipsychotics include:

- Risperidone

- Olanzapine

- Quetiapine

- Ziprasidone

- Aripiprazole

- Paliperidone

- Lurasidone

According to a research review by the Agency for Healthcare Research and Quality (AHRQ), typical and atypical antipsychotics both work to treat symptoms of schizophrenia and the manic phase of bipolar disorder.

Several atypical antipsychotics have a "broader spectrum" of action than the older medications, and are used for treating bipolar depression or depression that has not responded to an antidepressant medication alone.

How Do People Respond To Antipsychotics?

Certain symptoms, such as feeling agitated and having hallucinations, usually go away within days of starting an antipsychotic medication. Symptoms like delusions usually go away within a few weeks, but the full effects of the medication may not be seen for up to six weeks. Every patient responds differently, so it may take several trials of different antipsychotic medications to find the one that works best.

Some people may have a relapse—meaning their symptoms come back or get worse. Usually relapses happen when people stop taking their medication, or when they only take it sometimes. Some people stop taking the medication because they feel better or they may feel that they don't need it anymore, but no one should stop taking an antipsychotic medication without talking to his or her doctor. When a doctor says it is okay to stop taking a medication, it should be gradually tapered off—never stopped suddenly. Many people must stay on an antipsychotic continuously for months or years in order to stay well; treatment should be personalized for each individual.

What Are The Possible Side Effects Of Antipsychotics?

Antipsychotics have many side effects (or adverse events) and risks. The FDA lists the following side effects of antipsychotic medicines:

- drowsiness
- dizziness
- restlessness
- weight gain (the risk is higher with some atypical antipsychotic medicines)
- dry mouth
- constipation
- nausea

- vomiting

- blurred vision

- low blood pressure

- uncontrollable movements, such as tics and tremors (the risk is higher with typical anti-psychotic medicines)

- seizures

- a low number of white blood cells, which fight infections

A person taking an atypical antipsychotic medication should have his or her weight, glucose levels, and lipid levels monitored regularly by a doctor.

Typical antipsychotic medications can also cause additional side effects related to physical movement, such as:

- rigidity

- persistent muscle spasms

- tremors

- restlessness

Long-term use of typical antipsychotic medications may lead to a condition called tardive dyskinesia (TD). TD causes muscle movements, commonly around the mouth, that a person can't control. TD can range from mild to severe, and in some people, the problem cannot be cured. Sometimes people with TD recover partially or fully after they stop taking typical antipsychotic medication. People who think that they might have TD should check with their doctor before stopping their medication. TD rarely occurs while taking atypical antipsychotics.

Antipsychotics may cause other side effects that are not included in this list above.

Mood Stabilizers

Mood stabilizers are used primarily to treat bipolar disorder, mood swings associated with other mental disorders, and in some cases, to augment the effect of other medications used to treat depression. Lithium, which is an effective mood stabilizer, is approved for the treatment of mania and the maintenance treatment of bipolar disorder. A number of cohort studies describe anti-suicide benefits of lithium for individuals on long-term maintenance.

Mood stabilizers work by decreasing abnormal activity in the brain and are also sometimes used to treat:

- depression (usually along with an antidepressant)
- schizoaffective disorder
- disorders of impulse control
- certain mental illnesses in children

Anticonvulsant medications are also used as mood stabilizers. They were originally developed to treat seizures, but they were found to help control unstable moods as well. One anticonvulsant commonly used as a mood stabilizer is valproic acid (also called divalproex sodium). For some people, especially those with "mixed" symptoms of mania and depression or those with rapid-cycling bipolar disorder, valproic acid may work better than lithium. Other anticonvulsants used as mood stabilizers include:

- Carbamazepine
- Lamotrigine
- Oxcarbazepine

What Are The Possible Side Effects Of Mood Stabilizers?

Mood stabilizers can cause several side effects, and some of them may become serious, especially at excessively high blood levels. These side effects include:

- itching, rash
- excessive thirst
- frequent urination
- tremor (shakiness) of the hands
- nausea and vomiting
- slurred speech
- fast, slow, irregular, or pounding heartbeat
- blackouts
- changes in vision
- seizures

- hallucinations (seeing things or hearing voices that do not exist)

- loss of coordination

- swelling of the eyes, face, lips, tongue, throat, hands, feet, ankles, or lower legs.

If a person with bipolar disorder is being treated with lithium, he or she should visit the doctor regularly to check the lithium levels his or her blood, and make sure the kidneys and the thyroid are working normally.

Lithium is eliminated from the body through the kidney, so the dose may need to be lowered in older people with reduced kidney function. Also, loss of water from the body, such as through sweating or diarrhea, can cause the lithium level to rise, requiring a temporary lowering of the daily dose. Although kidney functions are checked periodically during lithium treatment, actual damage of the kidney is uncommon in people whose blood levels of lithium have stayed within the therapeutic range.

Mood stabilizers may cause other side effects that are not included in this list.

Some possible side effects linked to anticonvulsants (such as valproic acid) include:

- drowsiness

- dizziness

- headache

- diarrhea

- constipation

- changes in appetite

- weight changes

- back pain

- agitation

- mood swings

- abnormal thinking

- uncontrollable shaking of a part of the body

- loss of coordination

- uncontrollable movements of the eyes

- blurred or double vision

- ringing in the ears

- hair loss

These medications may also:

- cause damage to the liver or pancreas, so people taking it should see their doctors regularly

- increase testosterone (a male hormone) levels in teenage girls and lead to a condition called polycystic ovarian syndrome (a disease that can affect fertility and make the menstrual cycle become irregular)

Medications for common adult health problems, such as diabetes, high blood pressure, anxiety, and depression may interact badly with anticonvulsants. In this case, a doctor can offer other medication options.

Chapter 30
Technology And The Future Of Mental Health Treatment

Current Trends in App Development

Technology has opened a new frontier in mental health support and data collection. Mobile devices like cell phones, smartphones, and tablets are giving the public, doctors, and researchers new ways to access help, monitor progress, and increase understanding of mental wellbeing.

Mobile mental health support can be very simple but effective. For example, anyone with the ability to send a text message can contact a crisis center. New technology can also be packaged into an extremely sophisticated app for smartphones or tablets. Such apps might use the device's built-in sensors to collect information on a user's typical behavior patterns. If the app detects a change in behavior, it may provide a signal that help is needed before a crisis occurs. Some apps are stand-alone programs that promise to improve memory or thinking skills. Others help the user connect to a peer counselor or to a healthcare professional.

Excitement about the huge range of opportunities has led to a burst of app development. There are thousands of mental health apps available in iTunes and Android app stores, and the number is growing every year. However, this new technology frontier includes a lot of uncertainty. There is very little industry regulation and very little information on app effectiveness, which can lead consumers to wonder which apps they should trust.

Before focusing on the state of the science and where it may lead, it's important to look at the advantages and disadvantages of expanding mental health treatment and research into a mobile world.

About This Chapter: This chapter includes text excerpted from "Technology And The Future Of Mental Health Treatment," National Institute of Mental Health (NIMH), May 2016.

The Pros and Cons Of Mental Health Apps

Experts believe that technology has a lot of potential for clients and clinicians alike. A few of the advantages of mobile care include:

- **Convenience:** Treatment can take place anytime and anywhere (e.g., at home in the middle of the night or on a bus on the way to work) and may be ideal for those who have trouble with in-person appointments.

- **Anonymity:** Clients can seek treatment options without involving other people.

- **An introduction to care:** Technology may be a good first step for those who have avoided mental healthcare in the past.

- **Lower cost:** Some apps are free or cost less than traditional care.

- **Service to more people:** Technology can help mental health providers offer treatment to people in remote areas or to many people in times of sudden need (for example, following a natural disaster or terror attack).

- **Interest:** Some technologies might be more appealing than traditional treatment methods, which may encourage clients to continue therapy.

- **24-hour service:** Technology can provide round-the-clock monitoring or intervention support.

- **Consistency:** Technology can offer the same treatment program to all users.

- **Support:** Technology can complement traditional therapy by extending an in-person session, reinforcing new skills, and providing support and monitoring.

This new era of mental health technology offers great opportunities but also raises a number of concerns. Tackling potential problems will be an important part of making sure new apps provide benefits without causing harm. That is why the mental health community and software developers are focusing on:

- **Effectiveness:** The biggest concern with technological interventions is obtaining scientific evidence that they work and that they work as well as traditional methods.

- **For whom and for what:** Another concern is understanding if apps work for all people and for all mental health conditions.

- **Guidance:** There are no industry-wide standards to help consumers know if an app or other mobile technology is proven effective.

- **Privacy:** Apps deal with very sensitive personal information so app makers need to be able to guarantee privacy for app users.

- **Regulation:** The question of who will or should regulate mental health technology and the data it generates needs to be answered.

- **Overselling:** There is some concern that if an app or program promises more than it delivers, consumers may turn away from other, more effective therapies.

Current Trends in App Development

Creative research and engineering teams are combining their skills to address a wide range of mental health concerns. Some popular areas of app development include:

Self-Management Apps

"Self-management" means that the user puts information into the app so that the app can provide feedback. For example, the user might set up medication reminders, or use the app to develop tools for managing stress, anxiety, or sleep problems. Some software can use additional equipment to track heart rate, breathing patterns, blood pressure, etc., and may help the user track progress and receive feedback.

Apps for Improving Thinking Skills

Apps that help the user with cognitive remediation (improved thinking skills) are promising. These apps are often targeted toward people with serious mental illnesses.

Skill-Training Apps

Skill-training apps may feel more like games than other mental health apps as they help users learn new coping or thinking skills. The user might watch an educational video about anxiety management or the importance of social support. Next, the user might pick some new strategies to try and then use the app to track how often those new skills are practiced.

Illness Management, Supported Care

This type of app technology adds additional support by allowing the user to interact with another human being. The app may help the user connect with peer support or may send information to a trained healthcare provider who can offer guidance and therapy options. Researchers are working to learn how much human interaction people need for app-based treatments to be effective.

Passive Symptom Tracking

A lot of effort is going into developing apps that can collect data using the sensors built into smartphones. These sensors can record movement patterns, social interactions (such as the number of texts and phone calls), behavior at different times of the day, vocal tone and speed, and more. In the future, apps may be able to analyze these data to determine the user's real-time state of mind. Such apps may be able to recognize changes in behavior patterns that signal a mood episode such as mania, depression, or psychosis before it occurs. An app may not replace a mental health professional, but it may be able to alert caregivers when a client needs additional attention. The goal is to create apps that support a range of users, including those with serious mental illnesses.

Data Collection

Data collection apps can gather data without any help from the user. Receiving information from a large number of individuals at the same time can increase researchers' understanding of mental health and help them develop better interventions.

Evaluating Apps

There are no review boards, checklists, or widely accepted rules for choosing a mental health app. Most apps do not have peer-reviewed research to support their claims, and it is unlikely that every mental health app will go through a randomized, controlled research trial to test effectiveness. One reason is that testing is a slow process and technology evolves quickly. By the time an app has been put through rigorous scientific testing, the original technology may be outdated.

Currently, there are no national standards for evaluating the effectiveness of the hundreds of mental health apps that are available. Consumers should be cautious about trusting a program. However, there are a few suggestions for finding an app that may work for you:

- Ask a trusted healthcare provider for a recommendation. Some larger providers may offer several apps and collect data on their use.

- Check to see if the app offers recommendations for what to do if symptoms get worse or if there is a psychiatric emergency.

- Decide if you want an app that is completely automated or an app that offers opportunities for contact with a trained person.

- Search for information on the app developer. Can you find helpful information about his or her credentials and experience?

- Beware of misleading logos. The National Institute of Mental Health (NIMH) has not developed and does not endorse any apps. However, some app developers have unlawfully used the NIMH logo to market their products.

- Search the PubMed database offered by National Library of Medicine (www.ncbi.nlm.nih.gov/pubmed). This resource contains articles on a wide range of research topics, including mental health app development.

- If there is no information about a particular app, check to see if it is based on a treatment that has been tested. For example, research has shown that Internet-based cognitive behavior therapy (CBT) is as effective as conventional CBT for disorders that respond well to CBT, like depression, anxiety, social phobia, and panic disorder.

- Try it. If you're interested in an app, test it for a few days and decide if it's easy to use, holds your attention, and if you want to continue using it. An app is only effective if keeps users engaged for weeks or months.

Chapter 31

Understanding Drug Use And Addiction

Many people don't understand why or how other people become addicted to drugs. They may mistakenly think that those who use drugs lack moral principles or willpower and that they could stop their drug use simply by choosing to. In reality, drug addiction is a complex disease, and quitting usually takes more than good intentions or a strong will. Drugs change the brain in ways that make quitting hard, even for those who want to. Fortunately, researchers know more than ever about how drugs affect the brain and have found treatments that can help people recover from drug addiction and lead productive lives.

What Is Drug Addiction?

Addiction is a chronic disease characterized by drug seeking and use that is compulsive, or difficult to control, despite harmful consequences. The initial decision to take drugs is voluntary for most people, but repeated drug use can lead to brain changes that challenge an addicted person's self-control and interfere with their ability to resist intense urges to take drugs. These brain changes can be persistent, which is why drug addiction is considered a "relapsing" disease—people in recovery from drug use disorders are at increased risk for returning to drug use even after years of not taking the drug.

It's common for a person to relapse, but relapse doesn't mean that treatment doesn't work. As with other chronic health conditions, treatment should be ongoing and should be adjusted based on how the patient responds. Treatment plans need to be reviewed often and modified to fit the patient's changing needs.

About This Chapter: This chapter includes text excerpted from "DrugFacts—Understanding Drug Use And Addiction," National Institute on Drug Abuse (NIDA), August 2016.

What Happens To The Brain When A Person Takes Drugs?

Most drugs affect the brain's "reward circuit" by flooding it with the chemical messenger dopamine. This reward system controls the body's ability to feel pleasure and motivates a person to repeat behaviors needed to thrive, such as eating and spending time with loved ones. This overstimulation of the reward circuit causes the intensely pleasurable "high" that can lead people to take a drug again and again.

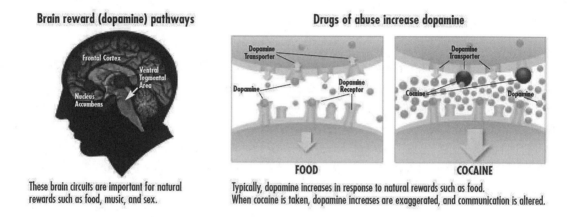

Brain reward (dopamine) pathways

These brain circuits are important for natural rewards such as food, music, and sex.

Drugs of abuse increase dopamine

FOOD   COCAINE

Typically, dopamine increases in response to natural rewards such as food.
When cocaine is taken, dopamine increases are exaggerated, and communication is altered.

Figure 31.1. Drugs Of Abuse Target The Brain's Pleasure Center

As a person continues to use drugs, the brain adjusts to the excess dopamine by making less of it and/or reducing the ability of cells in the reward circuit to respond to it. This reduces the high that the person feels compared to the high they felt when first taking the drug—an effect known as tolerance. They might take more of the drug, trying to achieve the same dopamine high. It can also cause them to get less pleasure from other things they once enjoyed, like food or social activities.

Long-term use also causes changes in other brain chemical systems and circuits as well, affecting functions that include:

- learning
- judgment
- decision-making
- stress

- memory

- behavior

Despite being aware of these harmful outcomes, many people who use drugs continue to take them, which is the nature of addiction.

Teens, Depression And Marijuana

According to a report by Office of National Drug Control Policy (ONDCP) on teens, depression and marijuana use:

- Depressed teens are twice as likely as non-depressed teens to use marijuana and other illicit drugs.
- Depressed teens are more than twice as likely as their peers to abuse or become dependent on marijuana.
- Marijuana use can worsen depression and lead to more serious mental illness such as schizophrenia, anxiety, and even suicide.
- Teens who smoke marijuana at least once a month are three times more likely to have suicidal thoughts than non-users.
- The percentage of depressed teens is equal to the percentage of depressed adults, but depressed teens are more likely than depressed adults to use marijuana than other drugs.

(Source: "The Dangers And Consequences Of Marijuana Abuse," Drug Enforcement Administration (DEA).)

Why Do Some People Become Addicted To Drugs While Others Don't?

No one factor can predict if a person will become addicted to drugs. A combination of factors influences risk for addiction. The more risk factors a person has, the greater the chance that taking drugs can lead to addiction. For example:

- **Biology.** The genes that people are born with account for about half of a person's risk for addiction. Gender, ethnicity, and the presence of other mental disorders may also influence risk for drug use and addiction.

- **Environment.** A person's environment includes many different influences, from family and friends to economic status and general quality of life. Factors such as peer pressure, physical and sexual abuse, early exposure to drugs, stress, and parental guidance can greatly affect a person's likelihood of drug use and addiction.

- **Development.** Genetic and environmental factors interact with critical developmental stages in a person's life to affect addiction risk. Although taking drugs at any age can lead to addiction, the earlier that drug use begins, the more likely it will progress to addiction. This is particularly problematic for teens. Because areas in their brains that control decision-making, judgment, and self-control are still developing, teens may be especially prone to risky behaviors, including trying drugs.

Can Drug Addiction Be Cured Or Prevented?

As with most other chronic diseases, such as diabetes, asthma, or heart disease, treatment for drug addiction generally isn't a cure. However, addiction is treatable and can be successfully managed. People who are recovering from an addiction will be at risk for relapse for years and possibly for their whole lives. Research shows that combining addiction treatment medicines with behavioral therapy ensures the best chance of success for most patients. Treatment approaches tailored to each patient's drug use patterns and any co-occurring medical, mental, and social problems can lead to continued recovery.

More good news is that drug use and addiction are preventable. Results from National Institute on Drug Abuse (NIDA) funded research have shown that prevention programs involving families, schools, communities, and the media are effective for preventing or reducing drug use and addiction. Although personal events and cultural factors affect drug use trends, when young people view drug use as harmful, they tend to decrease their drug taking. Therefore, education and outreach are key in helping people understand the possible risks of drug use. Teachers, parents, and healthcare providers have crucial roles in educating young people and preventing drug use and addiction.

Chapter 32
Moving Towards A Hopeful Future

Many survivors talk about a "second chance," or slowly coming to value what would have been lost if their attempt had resulted in their death. Over time, they begin to reclaim a sense of purpose in their lives, a new sense of identity, and real reasons for hope.

When you made your suicide attempt, you felt as if suicide was a way to end your pain. At that moment, in your mind, your reasons for dying outweighed your reasons for living. As you've learned, reconnecting with your reasons for living can help you build hope. Some survivors recommend putting together a "hope box" that can serve as a physical reminder of the things in your life that bring you joy. When you begin to feel bad about yourself or your life and feel depressed, the contents of your hope box can help lift your spirits. It also is a good place to keep your safety plan.

Staying In Control By Being Organized

Dealing with stress or emotional pain can feel overwhelming and lead you to neglect day-to-day tasks and responsibilities. Feeling like life is out of control can make anyone feel anxious. It might help to make a list of the things you have to do each day. That way, you won't forget important events or get distracted and not complete things you need to get done.

Checking items off a to-do list can also help you feel a sense of accomplishment. Keep it simple and short to begin with; you can always add more when you have more energy. Keeping a calendar and using a daily planner are great ways to help yourself stay organized and maintain a sense of control over your life.

About This Chapter: This chapter includes text excerpted from "A Journey Toward Health And Hope," Substance Abuse and Mental Health Services Administration (SAMHSA), 2015.

Creating A Hope Box

Your hope box can contain anything that might help you put aside painful thoughts or negative emotions and instead remind you of things in life that you enjoy. Decorating the box can be fun, as well. Here are some ideas for things to include:

- Photos or letters from people you care about.
- Poems, books, or scripture passages that lift you up.
- Movies or music you like.
- Note cards with uplifting words or thoughts, things that have kept you going in the past, or memories of happy times.
- Special trinkets or mementos that help you feel grounded.
- Your safety plan.

Your box can contain actual objects or be a collection of links or digital files on your computer, cell phone, e-reader, or other device.

Getting In Touch With Your Spirituality

Some suicide attempt survivors find comfort in spirituality. Spirituality can mean different things to different people, and for some it can provide a feeling of being connected to something larger than themselves. Some may experience this by attending churches, temples, synagogues, mosques, and other places of worship. Others discover deeper meanings in nature, philosophy, or music. Would getting in touch with your spirituality bring you comfort and peace? Only you can answer that, but it does help some people.

Maintaining A Healthy Lifestyle

Maintaining a healthy lifestyle can affect the way you feel, not only physically, but emotionally. If you feel depressed or overwhelmed emotionally, it's easy to forget the basics of taking care of yourself physically. It will make a difference if you maintain a healthy lifestyle during your recovery. Of course this means limiting your use of alcohol and eliminating other drugs, as these can negatively affect your emotions, but it's more than just that. Getting enough sleep, eating well, and exercising are also crucial to your recovery.

Sleep

A link between sleep and depression is well-documented. When depressed, many people find themselves sleeping a lot more than usual, while others are unable to sleep adequately.

Poor sleep can lead to fatigue, inactivity, anxiety, and irritability, making depression or other mental health issues even worse. Insomnia can also be associated with suicidal thoughts and actions. If you have depression that includes sleep disturbances, certain kinds of talk therapy (like CBT) can help, as well as medication. So it is important to discuss sleep problems with your counselor or psychiatrist.

Getting enough sleep is crucial because your body restores itself during sleep.

Diet

Appetite changes—either poor appetite with weight loss or increased appetite with weight gain—also can be symptoms of major depression. If your appetite has changed and you have low, depressed mood, please talk with your psychiatrist or counselor about whether you should consider medication.

While no particular diet has been proven to decrease depression and anxiety or improve emotional health, there does seem to be a correlation between what we eat and how we feel. A healthy diet is recommended as a key part of the overall treatment for depression. Additionally, ensuring that your body has the nutrients it needs can increase your energy level.

Enrolling in a healthy cooking class can help you find ways to eat well and meet new people. You also can find out how to prepare healthy food online.

Exercise

When you exercise, your body releases endorphins, a chemical that affects how people perceive pain. It's believed that the release of endorphins can help people feel more energized and even improve their emotional states, allowing them to be more hopeful about life. In fact, some studies suggest that exercise can be an effective treatment for depression.

Given that exercise can improve your mood, you might want to join a local gym, take a walk every day with a friend, or do exercises at home. Incorporating an exercise plan into your daily life (exercising three or more times each week) is highly recommended. You can find more information about depression and exercise online.

Taking Medication

If you choose to go to counseling, your counselor may recommend taking medication to improve your mood, especially if maintaining a healthy lifestyle and counseling aren't giving you the results you're looking for. You may struggle with the decision to take medication and feel as though it's a sign of weakness. It's important to remember that people take medications for all sorts of illnesses, and there is no reason to be embarrassed if you choose to try medications to alleviate depression, anxiety, or another mental health concern that causes you pain.

Certainly, only you can decide if you want to take medication; however, many people have felt that their depression and anxiety improved after taking medication. Most people (including researchers) indicate that counseling combined with medication provides the best results.

If you do choose to try medication, here are a few important things to remember:

- It can take some time for medication to have an effect. While some medications (for instance, sleep medication) may work immediately, medications for depression may take up to 8 weeks to reach their full effect. Your psychiatrist or doctor can tell you what to expect.

- You must take your medication as directed, without skipping dosages, for it to be effective.

- It's important to continue taking your medication for the entire period it is prescribed. You may be tempted to stop taking medication when you start to feel better. Stopping too soon can cause a relapse. Always work with your psychiatrist or doctor if you want to stop or change your medication.

- If your thoughts of suicide increase after you start taking medication, be sure to contact your psychiatrist or doctor immediately.

- Different medications work for different people. Be patient; sometimes it can take time to find the medications that work best for you. If one medication doesn't work, that doesn't mean none of them will. Finding the right medication can take persistence.

Advocating For Others To Support Your Recovery

When you're feeling stronger, you may find that helping others who are facing suicide can help you, too. Sharing your experiences and wisdom might save other lives. And saving lives can be a source of pride and accomplishment for you. Speaking about your experience also helps to break the guilt and shame that can be associated with suicide and lets others know they're not alone.

You should give serious consideration to whether you're ready to talk openly about your suicide attempt before deciding to advocate for others. It's important to ensure that you've given yourself enough time to heal and learn from your experience before using it to help others. Some questions you might ask yourself include:

- Am I ready to speak? Have I healed enough to speak?

- Am I prepared for my family's reactions to going public?

- Am I prepared for the possible social effects of going public with my story?

- Am I familiar with the resources available to help others?

- How will I take care of myself?

Some ways to help others when the time is right include:

- Becoming a member of a national organization that advocates for suicide prevention

- Helping raise funds for suicide prevention

- Participating in a suicide prevention walk

- Volunteering at a crisis hotline

- Organizing an attempt survivors' support group

- Writing or talking with others about your journey to raise public awareness about suicide and recovery

Hopes For A Safe Journey

The time after your suicide attempt is an important one. It can be a turning point in your life. Often, your suicide attempt can break the silence that surrounded the problems you were experiencing and your suicidal thoughts. Making a choice to be open about how you're feeling and seeking help, when you're ready, can be the first step on the path to a more fulfilling life.

As discussed, recovering from your suicide attempt is a process. It will likely have its ups and downs. You may feel overwhelmed or sad at times, and you may experience suicidal thoughts again. However, it's important to remember that feelings change. Finding ways to cope with those negative feelings while staying alive will give you a chance to enjoy the positive things life has in store for you.

Always remember:

- You are not alone.

- You matter.

- Life can get better.

- It may be difficult, but the effort you invest in your recovery will be worth it.

201

Part Four
When Someone You Know Dies From Suicide

Chapter 33
Surviving Suicide Loss

Death By Suicide

The end of life can come by many means. But suicide is the most complicated for those left behind. Why?

Suicide is violent, but so is homicide. It's swift and doesn't leave time for closure, but so is a fatal car crash. Death by suicide can encompass all these characteristics.

Where suicide differs from other deaths is inherent in the act. Suicide is a deliberate end to life that most of us could not consider. It doesn't seem possible that someone could engage in such behavior. Could life be so bad someone could extinguish it forever?

Perhaps answers lie in what can bring someone to the brink of suicide. Research has shown that about 60 percent of youth and about 90 percent of adults who die by suicide had a mental illness and/or alcohol or substance use disorder.

The problem is, these disorders often go unrecognized or untreated. People may grapple with explosive anger, anxiety attacks, debilitating depression or mood swings, but they, and those close to them, may not recognize these behaviors as treatable or changeable.

Also, alcoholism and/or substance use disorders and other addictions are often present in those who die by suicide and who use these substances to self-medicate what's been called the unrelenting "psychache" they feel.

Bottom line? People who die by suicide don't necessarily want to die. On the contrary, they feel they must end the intense and ongoing pain of living.

About This Chapter: This chapter includes text excerpted from "Supporting Survivors Of Suicide Loss," Substance Abuse and Mental Health Services Administration (SAMHSA), February 2009. Reviewed January 2017.

Sudden Loss

What Survivors Feel

Death of a loved one by suicide can be jolting and unforgiving. The impact on those closest to the deceased—parent, sibling, spouse, child, friend—can be profound and long lasting. People close to the deceased are known as "survivors" of suicide loss. It may be challenging for survivors to cope and function in the days to come. They may compartmentalize their grief and keep it in a place deep within themselves. Most are changed by such a traumatic death.

Questions can preoccupy survivors of suicide loss. These questions may be incessant, and can be part of coping with suicide loss. They can lead survivors to assume guilt in bearing responsibility for another's death. This level of responsibility—perceived or actual—is often not as common when death comes about by other means.

When someone fails to recognize potential for suicide in one closest to them, they feel exposed and vulnerable to their core. Feelings of incompetence in other aspects of their lives may rise to the surface. These perceptions of self, while often distorted, can be intensified by societal response to suicide, and the stigma it brings.

"What did you miss?" "What a coward." "How could he do this to you?" "What a waste." They may be spoken with an overtone of concern for the bereaved, yet they signal stigma and shame. Comments such as these intensify the grief and guilt already burdened upon the bereaved by the abrupt loss of their loved one.

Suicide: A Sin?

Some view suicide as a sin, one that may condemn a person. The anguish that can precede suicide is incomprehensible to most of us. Prior to death, the deceased's judgment may be clouded by mental illness, alcohol or tunnel vision that can distort rational thought. In recent years many faith communities have come to accept suicide as the tragic outcome of mental illness. Yet many in society still consider suicide as a sin, thus perpetuating this stigmatizing view of an act that is frequently based in mental illness.

Stigma Of Suicide

Subtle Messages In Mere Words

Few issues in society are as stigma laden as suicide. This stigma is intensified, say experts, by language commonly used to describe suicidal people and gestures. Experts suggest choosing words with care when talking with those who have had a loss to suicide to minimize stigma. Consider the following:

"She committed suicide."

The word "commit" implies something morally wrong, as in the religious concept of committing a sin or crime. Yet research shows that about 60 percent of youth and about 90 percent of adults who die by suicide have an underlying mental and/or alcohol or substance use disorder that is not their fault, just as cancer or heart disease is not the fault of those who die from these illnesses.

Better choice: "She completed suicide" or "She died by suicide."

"He attempted suicide before he succeeded."

We succeed at good things in life—education, relationships, skills and hobbies. So to say someone "succeeded" at killing themselves is inappropriate in its positive implications for a tragic act.

Better choice: "He died by suicide after a prior attempt."

"Sometimes people make poor choices."

We wouldn't say that someone who died from cancer made poor choices. The same goes for suicide. Research has shown that people who die by suicide see no other way. Many do not want to die, but succumb to the excruciating pain of living. To them, in the midst of mental illness or overwhelming anxiety, loss or hopelessness, the decision to die is not about "choice" but escaping pain. To call suicide a choice—and a poor one at that—minimizes the extreme suffering that preceded it.

Better choice: "Life is so unfair."

"What a waste. How selfish of him."

Many people who die by suicide may have struggled against incredible odds, perhaps for years. Their last act may seem a response to an emotional blow such as job loss, end of a relationship, health diagnosis or brush with the law. Yet for many, an underlying mental or alcohol and/or substance use disorder has made them vulnerable to suicide. These disorders can bring distress, anguish, and despair. To call suicide a waste or a selfish act makes light of the complexity of this loss and events leading up to it.

Better choice "What a tragedy."

"Don't feel guilty. You did all you could."

Telling survivors of suicide loss not to feel guilty can be futile, no matter how good your intentions. Moreover, your efforts to ease survivors' guilt can run counter to their instincts. Loved ones may think they have not done all they could for the person who died by suicide. They may need to work through those feelings on their own or with a mental health professional. Telling survivors not to feel the guilt they're already experiencing may make them feel worse because their feelings are being dismissed or diminished, not acknowledged and accepted by others. Instead, giving survivors permission to be where they're emotionally at can be a gift.

Better choice "I'm here to support you wherever you are at."

Turbulent Emotions Of Suicide Loss

As after other deaths, those left in the wake of suicide feel a multitude of emotions such as denial, fear, anger and abandonment. Suicide can heighten these feelings or bring others such as:

Anguish

"I feel a palpable pain in my heart, so profound that it's a physical ache."

Guilt

If only I would have not gone to work that day, he would still be alive."

Betrayal

"We were supposed to be in this together—be there for one another. But she abandoned me to deal with the awful aftermath of all this."

Relief

"Living with him was so hard. I have a sense of relief that he isn't suffering anymore, but I feel incredibly guilty about being relieved that he's dead."

Incompetence

"I'm supposed to protect my loved ones. But she wanted out so bad that I couldn't even protect her from herself."

Ills That Can Accompany Suicide Loss

- Exhaustion

- Migraines

- Posttraumatic stress disorder

- Memory problems

- Colitis

- Alcoholism

- Sleep problems

- Anxiety

- Crying spells

- Heart trouble

- Fear of being alone

- Ulcers

- Difficulty with relationships

- Clinical depression

- Thoughts of suicide

Relief May Be Real

Those who succumb to suicide may have placed heavy emotional and financial burdens on loved ones prior to death. So there may be a sense of relief when this person passes, a feeling that "perhaps this was for the best" and the deceased is at peace.

Chapter 34
Understanding Grief, Bereavement, And Mourning

Bereavement And Grief

Bereavement is the period of sadness after losing a loved one through death.

Grief and mourning occur during the period of bereavement. Grief and mourning are closely related. Mourning is the way we show grief in public. The way people mourn is affected by beliefs, religious practices, and cultural customs. People who are grieving are sometimes described as bereaved.

Grief is the normal process of reacting to the loss.

Grief is the emotional response to the loss of a loved one. Common grief reactions include the following:

- Feeling emotionally numb.

- Feeling unable to believe the loss occurred.

- Feeling anxiety from the distress of being separated from the loved one.

- Mourning along with depression.

- A feeling of acceptance.

About This Chapter: This chapter includes text excerpted from "Grief, Bereavement, And Coping With Loss (PDQ®)—Patient Version," National Cancer Institute (NCI), March 6, 2013. Reviewed January 2017.

> **Bereavement** is the state of having lost a significant other to death.
>
> **Grief** is the personal response to the loss.
>
> **Mourning** is the public expression of that loss.
>
> *(Source: "Bereavement, Grief, And Mourning," Mental Illness Research, Education and Clinical Center (MIRECC), U.S. Department of Veterans Affairs (VA))*

Types Of Grief Reactions

Normal Grief

Normal or common grief begins soon after a loss and symptoms go away over time.

During normal grief, the bereaved person moves toward accepting the loss and is able to continue normal day-to-day life even though it is hard to do. Common grief reactions include:

- Emotional numbness, shock, disbelief, or denial. These often occur right after the death, especially if the death was not expected.

- Anxiety over being separated from the loved one. The bereaved may wish to bring the person back and become lost in thoughts of the deceased. Images of death may occur often in the person's everyday thoughts.

- Distress that leads to crying; sighing; having dreams, illusions, and hallucinations of the deceased; and looking for places or things that were shared with the deceased.

- Anger.

- Periods of sadness, loss of sleep, loss of appetite, extreme tiredness, guilt, and loss of interest in life. Day-to-day living may be affected.

In normal grief, symptoms will occur less often and will feel less severe as time passes. Recovery does not happen in a set period of time. For most bereaved people having normal grief, symptoms lessen between 6 months and 2 years after the loss.

Many bereaved people will have grief bursts or pangs.

Grief bursts or pangs are short periods (20–30 minutes) of very intense distress. Sometimes these bursts are caused by reminders of the deceased person. At other times they seem to happen for no reason.

Grief is sometimes described as a process that has stages.

There are several theories about how the normal grief process works. Experts have described different types and numbers of stages that people go through as they cope with loss. At this time, there is not enough information to prove that one of these theories is more correct than the others.

Although many bereaved people have similar responses as they cope with their losses, there is no typical grief response. The grief process is personal.

Complicated Grief

There is no right or wrong way to grieve, but studies have shown that there are patterns of grief that are different from the most common. This has been called complicated grief.

Complicated grief reactions that have been seen in studies include:

- **Minimal grief reaction:** A grief pattern in which the person has no, or only a few, signs of distress or problems that occur with other types of grief.

- **Chronic grief:** A grief pattern in which the symptoms of common grief last for a much longer time than usual. These symptoms are a lot like ones that occur with major depression, anxiety, or posttraumatic stress.

Impact Of Suicide On Survivors

The grieving process is complex and unique for each survivor. Feelings may vary and can include shock, confusion, anger, guilt, relief, and sorrow. Questions to consider or things that may impact the grieving process include the following: What was the survivor's relationship with the deceased? Were they a caregiver? Who was their main source of support? Were they living with the member prior to the individual's death?

- **Guilt and confusion about responsibility:** Suicide is a confusing phenomenon, and when it occurs, it is not uncommon for those closest to the deceased to experience intense feelings of both guilt and blaming following the loss of a loved one. Family members may believe they should have recognized the signs their loved one was depressed or feel responsible for having encouraged the deceased to join the service in the first place.

- **Anger/blame:** In addition to such feelings of guilt, family members may look to externalize these emotions. These are normal responses suicide could be more pronounced if the circumstances around a loved one's suicide are unclear.

- **Mixed emotions and confusion:** Suicide can occur after a long period of emotional turmoil and/or persistent mental illness, both of which can have devastating effects on family members. Taking care of a loved one who has a serious mental illness can place considerable strain not only on the primary caregiver, but also on friends and other members of the family. If the survivor was closely involved with the deceased, it is likely that he or she felt significantly burdened, emotionally exhausted and at times helpless and scared. A sense of relief when a difficult situation ends is normal, but when the ending is suicide, feelings of relief may be unexpected and contribute to guilt and shame.

- **Vicarious trauma:** If violence and turmoil were prevalent in the home prior to the suicide (emotional abuse, physical abuse, domestic violence, substance use), family members are at risk for developing posttraumatic stress disorder (PTSD) and other emotional difficulties that may further complicate the grief process. For those who may be experiencing symptoms of posttraumatic stress or vicarious trauma while also dealing with the loss of a loved one, mental health treatment and additional support may be needed. Such individuals should be provided with resources and instructed to seek help if they begin to have thoughts of suicide or self-harm.

Helping Child Survivors

If the deceased was a parent or family member, talking to the children about the death may be one of the most difficult tasks you face. Suicide is a complicated form of death and requires honesty with children. However, the explanation provided should fit the child's age and level of understanding. If you're reluctant to talk to a child about suicide, what it means and why it happened, keep in mind that children are likely to hear it from other sources, which will lead to even more confusion, fear, and distress. Furthermore, talking to children can help erase misconceptions or concerns that somehow they are blame for what happened.

(Source: "Providing Support For Suicide Survivors: Understanding Pertinent Military/Veteran Issues," Mental Illness Research Education and Clinical Center (MIRECC), U.S. Department of Veterans Affairs (VA).)

Factors That Affect Complicated Grief

Researchers study grief reactions to try to find out what might increase the chance that complicated grief will occur.

Studies have looked at how the following factors affect the grief response:

Whether the death is expected or unexpected.

It may seem that any sudden, unexpected loss might lead to more difficult grief. However, studies have found that bereaved people with high self-esteem and/or a feeling that they have control over life are likely to have a normal grief reaction even after an unexpected loss. Bereaved people with low self-esteem and/or a sense that life cannot be controlled are more likely to have complicated grief after an unexpected loss. This includes more depression and physical problems.

The personality of the bereaved.

Studies have found that people with certain personality traits are more likely to have long-lasting depression after a loss. These include people who are very dependent on the loved one (such as a spouse), and people who deal with distress by thinking about it all the time.

The religious beliefs of the bereaved.

Some studies have shown that religion helps people cope better with grief. Other studies have shown it does not help or causes more distress. Religion seems to help people who go to church often. The positive effect on grief may be because churchgoers have more social support.

Whether the bereaved is male or female.

In general, men have more problems than women do after a spouse's death. Men tend to have worse depression and more health problems than women do after the loss. Some researchers think this may be because men have less social support after a loss.

The age of the bereaved.

In general, younger bereaved people have more problems after a loss than older bereaved people do. They have more severe health problems, grief symptoms, and other mental and physical symptoms. Younger bereaved people, however, may recover more quickly than older bereaved people do, because they have more resources and social support.

The amount of social support the bereaved has.

Lack of social support increases the chance of having problems coping with a loss. Social support includes the person's family, friends, neighbors, and community members who can give psychological, physical, and financial help. After the death of a close family member, many people have a number of related losses. The death of a spouse, for example, may cause a loss of income and changes in lifestyle and day-to-day living. These are all related to social support.

Children And Grief

Most children who have had a loss have three common worries about death.

Did I make the death happen?

Children often think that they have "magical powers." If a mother is irritated and says, "You'll be the death of me" and later dies, her child may wonder if he or she actually caused the mother's death. Also, when children argue, one may say (or think), "I wish you were dead." If that child dies, the surviving child may think that those thoughts caused the death.

Is it going to happen to me?

The death of another child may be very hard for a child. If the child thinks that the death may have been prevented (by either a parent or a doctor) the child may fear that he or she could also die.

Who is going to take care of me?

Since children depend on parents and other adults to take care of them, a grieving child may wonder who will care for him or her after the death of an important person.

Treatment Of Grief

Normal grief may not need to be treated.

Most bereaved people work through grief and recover within the first 6 months to 2 years. Researchers are studying whether bereaved people experiencing normal grief would be helped by formal treatment.

They are also studying whether treatment might prevent complicated grief in people who are likely to have it.

For people who have serious grief reactions or symptoms of distress, treatment may be helpful.

Complicated grief may be treated with different types of psychotherapy (talk therapy).

Researchers are studying the treatment of mental, emotional, social, and behavioral symptoms of grief. Treatment methods include discussion, listening, and counseling.

Complicated grief treatment (CGT) is a type of grief therapy that was helpful in a clinical trial.

Complicated grief treatment (CGT) has three phases:

- The first phase includes talking about the loss and setting goals toward recovery. The bereaved are taught to work on these two things.

- The second phase includes coping with the loss by retelling the story of the death. This helps bereaved people who try not to think about their loss.

- The last phase looks at progress that has been made toward recovery and helps the bereaved make future plans. The bereaved's feelings about ending the sessions are also discussed.

In a clinical trial of patients with complicated grief, CGT was compared to interpersonal psychotherapy (IPT). IPT is a type of psychotherapy that focuses on the person's relationships with others and is helpful in treating depression. In patients with complicated grief, the CGT was more helpful than IPT.

Cognitive behavioral therapy (CBT) for complicated grief was helpful in a clinical trial.

Cognitive behavioral therapy (CBT) works with the way a person's thoughts and behaviors are connected. CBT helps the patient learn skills that change attitudes and behaviors by replacing negative thoughts and changing the rewards of certain behaviors.

A clinical trial compared CBT to counseling for complicated grief. Results showed that patients treated with CBT had more improvement in symptoms and general mental distress than those in the counseling group.

Depression related to grief is sometimes treated with drugs.

There is no standard drug therapy for depression that occurs with grief. Some healthcare professionals think depression is a normal part of grief and doesn't need to be treated. Whether to treat grief-related depression with drugs is up to the patient and the healthcare professional to decide.

Clinical trials of antidepressants for depression related to grief have found that the drugs can help relieve depression. However, they give less relief and take longer to work than they do when used for depression that is not related to grief.

Chapter 35
Coping With Bereavement And Grief

Grief Tips

The following are many ideas to help people who are mourning a loved one's death. Different kinds of losses dictate different responses, so not all of these ideas will suit everyone. Likewise, no two people grieve alike—what works for one may not work for another. Treat this list for what it is; a gathering of assorted suggestions that various people have tried with success. Perhaps what helped them will help you. The emphasis here is on specific, practical ideas.

Talk regularly with a friend. Talking with another about what you think and feel is one of the best things you can do for yourself. It helps relieve some of the pressure you may feel, it can give you a sense of perspective, and it keeps you in touch with others. Look for someone who's a good listener and who has a caring soul. Then speak what's on your mind and in your heart. If this feels one-sided let that be okay for this period of your life. Chances are the other person will find meaning in what they're doing, and time will come when you'll have the chance to be a good listener for someone else. You'll be a better listener then, if you're a good talker now.

Walk. Go for walks outside every day if you can. Don't overdo it, but walk briskly enough that it feels invigorating. Sometimes try walking slowly enough so you can look carefully at what you see. Observe what nature has to offer you, what it can teach you. Enjoy as much as you are able to of the sights and sounds that come your way. If you like, walk with another person.

About This Chapter: This chapter includes text excerpted from "Bereavement, Grief, And Mourning," Mental Illness Research, Education and Clinical Center (MIRECC), U.S. Department of Veterans Affairs (VA), July 2013. Reviewed January 2017.

Carry or wear a linking object. Carry something in your pocket or purse that reminds you of the one who died—a keepsake they gave you perhaps, or small object they once carried or used or a memento you select for just this purpose. You might wear a piece of their jewelry in the same way. Whenever you want, reach for and gaze upon this object and remember what it signifies.

Visit the grave. Not all people prefer to do this. But if it feels right to you, then do so. Don't let others convince you this is a morbid thing to do. Spend whatever time feels right there. Stand or sit in the quietness and do what comes naturally: be silent or talk, breathe deeply or cry, recollect or pray. You may wish to add your distinctive touch to the gravesite—straighten it a bit, or add little signs of your love.

Create a memory book. Compile photographs, which document your loved one's life. Arrange them into some sort of order so they tell a story. Add other elements if you want: diplomas, newspaper clippings, awards, accomplishments, and reminders of significant events. Put all this in a special binder and keep it for other people to look at if they wish. Go through it on your own if you desire. Reminisce as you do so.

Recall your dreams. Your dreams often have important things to say about your feelings and about your relationship with the one who died. Your dreams may be scary or sad, especially early on. They may seem weird or crazy to you. You may find that your loved one appears in your dreams. Accept your dreams for what they are and see what you can learn from them. No one knows that better than you.

Tell people what helps you and what doesn't. People around you may not understand what you need. So tell them. If hearing your loved one's name spoken aloud by others feels good, say so. If you need more time alone, or assistance with chores you're unable to complete, or an occasional hug, be honest. People can't read your mind, so you'll have to speak it.

Write things down. Most people who are grieving become more forgetful than usual. So help yourself remember what you want by keeping track of it on paper or with whatever system works best for you. This may include writing down things you want to preserve about the person who has died.

Ask for a copy of the memorial service. If the funeral liturgy or memorial service holds special meaning for you because of what was spoken or read, ask for the words. Whoever participated in that ritual will feel gratified that what they prepared was appreciated. Turn to these words whenever you want. Some people find that these thoughts provide even more help weeks and months after the service.

Remember the serenity prayer. This prayer is attributed to theologian Reinhold Niebuhr, but it's actually an ancient German prayer. It has brought comfort and support to many that have suffered various kinds of afflictions. "God grant me the serenity to accept the things I cannot change; courage to change the things I can; and wisdom to know the difference."

Create a memory area at home. In a space that feels appropriate, arrange a small table that honors the person: a framed photograph or two, perhaps a prized possession or award or something they created or something they loved. This might be placed on a small table, a mantel or a desk. Some people like to use a grouping of candles, representing not just the person who died but others who have died as well. In that case a variety of candles can be arranged each representing a unique life.

Drink water. Grieving people can easily become dehydrated. Crying can naturally lead to that. And with your normal routines turned upside down, you may simply not drink as much or as regularly as you did before this death. Make this a way you care for yourself.

Use your hands. Sometimes there's value in doing repetitive things with your hands, something you don't have to think about very much because it becomes second nature. Knitting and crocheting are like that. So are carving, woodworking, polishing, solving jigsaw puzzles, painting, braiding, shoveling, washing, and countless other activities.

Give yourself respites from your grief. Just because you're grieving doesn't mean you must always be feeling sad or forlorn. There's value in sometimes consciously deciding that you'll think about something else for awhile, or that you'll do something you've always enjoyed doing. Sometimes this happens naturally and it's only later you realize that your grief has taken a back seat. Let it, this is not an indication you love that person any less or that you're forgetting them. It's a sign that you're human and you need relief from the unrelenting pressure. It can also be a healthy sign you're healing.

Create or commission a memory quilt. Sew or invite others to sew with you, or hire someone to sew for you. However you get it completed, put together a wall hanging or a bedroom quilt that remembers the important life events of the one who died. Take your time doing this. Make it what it is, a labor of love.

See a grief counselor. If you're concerned about how you're feeling and how well you're adapting make an appointment with a counselor who specializes in grief. Often you'll learn what you need both about grief and about yourself as a griever in only a few sessions. Ask questions of the counselor before you sign on. What specific training does he or she have? What accreditation? A person who is a family therapist or a psychologist doesn't necessarily understand the unique issues of someone in grief.

Begin your day with your loved one. If your grief is young, you'll probably wake up thinking of that person anyway. So why not decide that you'll include her or him from the start? Focus this time in a positive way. Bring to your mind fulfilling memories. Recall lessons that this person taught you, gifts he or she gave you. Think about how you can spend your day in ways that would be keeping in with your loved one's best self and with your best self. Then carry that best self with you through your day.

Invite someone to be your telephone buddy. If your grief and sadness hit you especially hard at times and you have no one nearby to turn to, ask someone you trust to be your telephone buddy. Ask their permission for you to call them whenever you feel you're at loose ends, day or night. Then put their number beside your phone and call them if you need them. Don't abuse the privilege, of course. And covenant that someday it will be payback time—someday you'll make yourself available to help someone else in the same way you've been helped. That will help you accept the care you're receiving.

Avoid certain people if you must. No one likes to be unfriendly or cold. But if there are people in your life who make it very difficult for you to do your grieving then do what you can to stay out of their way. Some people may lecture you or belittle you.

Donate their possessions meaningfully. Whether you give your loved one's personal possessions to someone you know or to a stranger, find ways to pass these things along so that others might benefit from them. Family members of friends might like to receive keepsakes. They or others might deserve tools, utensils, books or sporting equipment. Philanthropic organizations can put clothes to good use. Some wish to do this quickly following the death, while others wish to wait awhile.

Donate in the other's name. Honor the other's memory and spirit by giving a gift or gifts to a cause the other would appreciate. A favorite charity? A local fundraiser? A building project? Extend that person's influence even further.

Take a yoga class. People of almost any age can do yoga. More than conditioning your body, it helps you relax and focus your mind. It can be woven into a practice of meditation. It's a gentle art for that time in your life when you deserve gentleness all around you.

Connect on the Internet. If you're computer savvy, search the Internet. You'll find many resources for people in grief, as well as the opportunity to chat with fellow grievers. You can link up with others without leaving your home. You'll also find more to expand your horizons as a person who is beginning to grow.

Speak to a clergyperson. If you're searching for answers to the larger questions about life and death, religion, and spirituality, consider talking with a representative of your faith, or even another's faith. Consider becoming a spiritual friend with another and making your time of grieving a time of personal exploring.

Learn about your loved one from others. Listen to the stories others have to tell about the one, who died, stories you're familiar with and those you've never heard before. Spend time with their friends, schoolmates or colleagues. Invite them into your home. Solicit the writings of others. Preserve whatever you find out. Celebrate your time together.

Take a day off. When the mood is just right, take a one-day vacation. Do whatever you want, or don't do whatever you want. Travel somewhere or stay inside by yourself. Be very active or don't do anything at all. Just make it your day, whatever that means for you.

Invite someone to give you feedback. Select someone you trust, preferably someone familiar with the working of grief, to give you his or her reaction when you ask for it. If you want to check out how clearly you're thinking, how accurately you're remembering, how effectively you're coping, go to that person. Pose your questions, and then listen to their responses. What you choose to do with that information will be up to you.

Vent your anger rather than hold it in. You may feel awkward being angry when you're grieving, but anger is a common reaction. The expression holds true: anger is best out floating rather than in bloating. Even if you feel a bit ashamed as you do it, find ways to get it out of your system. Yell, even if it's in an empty house. Cry. Resist the temptation to be proper. Go for a brisk walk. Do a long, hard workout. Vacuum up a storm. Do some yard work. Physical activity helps release anger.

Give thanks every day. Whatever has happened to you, you still have things to be thankful for. Perhaps it's your memories, your remaining family, your support, your work; you own health—all sorts of things. Draw your attention to those parts of life that are worth appreciating, and then appreciate them.

Monitor signs of dependency. While it's normal to become more dependent upon others for awhile immediately after a death, it will not be helpful to continue in that role long term. Watch for signs that you're prolonging your need for assistance. Congratulate yourself when you do things for yourself.

Chapter 36
Trauma And The Grieving Teen

"Trauma" is often thought of as physical injuries. Psychological trauma is an emotionally painful, shocking, stressful, and sometimes life-threatening experience. It may or may not involve physical injuries, and can result from witnessing distressing events.

> **Traumatic Grief**
>
> Traumatic grief may include the death of a parent, primary caretaker, or sibling; or abrupt and/ or unexpected, accidental, or premature death or homicide of a close friend, family member, or other close relative.
>
> *(Source: "Types Of Trauma And Violence," Substance Abuse and Mental Health Services Administration (SAMHSA).)*

Reactions (responses) to trauma can be immediate or delayed. Reactions to trauma differ in severity and cover a wide range of behaviors and responses. Children with existing mental health problems, past traumatic experiences, and/or limited family and social supports may be more reactive to trauma. Frequently experienced responses among children after trauma are loss of trust and a fear of the event happening again.

It's important to remember:

- Children's reactions to trauma are strongly influenced by adults' responses to trauma.

- People from different cultures may have their own ways of reacting to trauma.

About This Chapter: This chapter includes text excerpted from "Helping Children And Adolescents Cope With Violence And Disasters: What Parents Can Do," National Institute of Mental Health (NIMH), 2015.

The Grieving Teen

Under ordinary circumstances, teenagers go through many changes in their body image, behavior, attachments, and feelings. Life becomes even more complex when a father, mother, or other significant person dies—a shattering experience faced by one child in every ten under age 18. While people in all age groups struggle with such losses, teenagers face particularly painful adjustments following the death of a loved one.

Do Teens Grieve Like Adults?

Teens grieve deeply, but often work very hard to hide their feelings. Fearing the vulnerability that comes with expression, they look for distractions rather than stay with the grief process long enough to find real relief. Teens can act as if nothing has happened while they are breaking up inside. You may observe teens who take on the role of caregiver to family members or friends, in effect denying their own grief. Young men of this age may have a particularly hard time when they have been taught that showing emotion is something that girls do, but macho guys don't.

Who Do Teens Trust And Talk To?

Teens often trust only their peers, believing that no one else can understand how they feel and how they react to life's problems. Relationships with friends can be deep and meaningful, sharing conflicts occurring at home and details of their love lives.

To gain the trust of teens, adults must become good, nonjudgmental listeners. Let teenagers know that you are interested in them, in their views, and in their ideas and thoughts. Let them know that you like and care for them. Support their ideas or gently introduce new ways to approach their ideas. Acknowledge their grief and offer your thoughts on how to ease their pain.

(Source: "Helping A Grieving Teen," Federal Occupational Health (FOH), U.S. Department of Health and Human Services (HHS).)

Commonly Experienced Responses To Trauma Among Adolescents

- Having flashbacks to the event (flashbacks are the mind reliving the event)
- Having nightmares or other sleep problems
- Avoiding reminders of the event
- Using or abusing drugs, alcohol, or tobacco
- Being disruptive, disrespectful, or behaving destructively

- Having physical complaints
- Feeling isolated or confused
- Being depressed
- Being angry
- Losing interest in fun activities
- Having suicidal thoughts.

Adolescents may feel guilty. They may feel guilt for not preventing injury or deaths. They also may have thoughts of revenge.

What Can Parents Do To Help?

After violence or disaster, parents and family members should identify and address their own feelings—this will allow them to help others. Explain to children what happened and let them know:

- you love them
- the event was not their fault
- you will do your best to take care of them
- it's okay for them to feel upset.

Do

- allow children to cry
- allow sadness
- let children talk about feelings
- let them write about feelings
- let them draw pictures about the event or their feelings.

Don't

- expect children to be brave or tough
- make children discuss the event before they are ready
- get angry if children show strong emotions

Other Tips

- If children have trouble sleeping give them extra attention, let them sleep with a light on, or let them sleep in your room (for a short time).

- Try to keep normal routines, for example, reading bedtime stories, eating dinner together, watching TV together, reading books, exercising, or playing games. If you can't keep normal routines, make new ones together.

- Help children feel in control when possible by letting them choose meals, pick out clothes, or make some decisions for themselves.

How Can I Help Young Children Who Experienced Trauma?

Helping children can start immediately, even at the scene of the event. Most children recover within a few weeks of a traumatic experience, while some may need help longer. Grief, a deep emotional response to loss, may take months to resolve. Children may experience grief over the loss of a loved one, teacher, friend, or pet. Grief may be re-experienced or worsened by news reports or the event's anniversary.

Some children may need help from a mental health professional. Some people may seek other kinds of help from community leaders. Identify children who need support and help them obtain it.

Examples of problematic behaviors could be:

- refusing to go to places that remind them of the event
- emotional numbness
- behaving dangerously
- unexplained anger/rage
- sleep problems including nightmares

Adult helpers should:

Pay attention to children.

- Listen to them.
- Accept/do not argue about their feelings.

It can be difficult to separate normal teen behavior from that of a grieving teen in trouble. Some of the indicators that let you know when a teen needs more than a help group or peer counselors are:

- dramatic behavior changes
- extraordinary pressure
- isolation
- depression
- death wish
- guilt
- substance abuse
- skipping school or dropping grades
- acting out sexually

(Source: "Helping A Grieving Teen," Federal Occupational Health (FOH), U.S. Department of Health and Human Services (HHS).)

- Help them cope with the reality of their experiences.

Reduce effects of other stressors, such as

- frequent moving or changes in place of residence
- long periods away from family and friends
- pressures to perform well in school
- transportation problems
- fighting within the family
- being hungry

Monitor healing.

- It takes time.
- Do not ignore severe reactions.
- Pay attention to sudden changes in behaviors, speech, language use, or strong emotions.

Remind children that adults

- love them

- support them

- will be with them when possible.

More About Trauma Stress

Some children will have prolonged mental health problems after a traumatic event. These may include grief, depression, anxiety, and posttraumatic stress disorder (PTSD). Some trauma survivors get better with some support. Others may need prolonged care from a mental health professional. If after a month in a safe environment children are not able to perform normal routines or new behavioral or emotional problems develop, then contact a health professional.

It's A Fact!!

Studies show that about 15 percent to 43 percent of girls and 14 percent to 43 percent of boys go through at least one trauma. Of those children and teens who have had a trauma, 3 percent to 15 percent of girls and 1 percent to 6 percent of boys develop PTSD. Rates of PTSD are higher for certain types of trauma survivors.

(Source: "PTSD In Children And Teens," U.S. Department of Veterans Affairs (VA).)

Support For A Grieving Teen

Does Peer Counseling Work?

Because teens are most open to fellow teens, one approach to providing help is through peers. And it works. Peer counseling is now an elective course in many schools for teens. Peer counselors are trained to look at all kinds of life problems on a personal level and then at ways to help their peers. They are introduced to different situations that may occur, and speakers are brought in to teach them about specific topics. Because teens are willing to listen to other teens, peer counseling can play an important role in establishing communication with distressed classmates and friends, as well as steering them to professional help if it is needed.

Do Grief Support Groups Work?

Another approach to dealing with grief is through grief support groups, and they work, too. By sharing feelings with one another, teens find out they are not alone and that others are also struggling to rebuild shattered lives. Grief groups help teens feel understood, accepted, and supported.

What Events Cause PTSD In Children?

Children and teens could have PTSD if they have lived through an event that could have caused them or someone else to be killed or badly hurt. Such events include sexual or physical abuse or other violent crimes. Disasters such as floods, school shootings, car crashes, or fires might also cause PTSD. Other events that can cause PTSD are war, a friend's suicide, or seeing violence in the area they live.

(Source: "PTSD In Children And Teens," U.S. Department of Veterans Affairs (VA).)

Chapter 37

How Suicide Affects Family Members

Someone I Know Has Died By Suicide

It is very upsetting when someone you know dies by suicide. Getting over the shock and distress will be especially hard if you felt close to them, if you saw the event, or if you have your own mental health issues.

Survivors
- A survivor of suicide is a family member or friend of a person who died by suicide.
- Surviving the loss of loved one to suicide is a risk factor for suicide.
- Surviving family members and close friends are deeply impacted by each suicide and experience a range of complex grief reactions including, guilt, anger, abandonment, denial, helplessness, and shock.
- No exact figure exists, but it is estimated that a median of between 6 and 32 survivors exist for each suicide, depending on the definition used.
- According to another estimate, approximately 7 percent of the U.S. population knew someone who died by suicide during the past 12 months.

(Source: "Suicide: Consequences," Centers for Disease Control and Prevention (CDC).)

Grieving the loss of a loved one is a natural process. It may take several months to feel "normal" again after someone you know dies by suicide. Due to the traumatic nature of suicide, you may go through what's known as "traumatic grief." If you are feeling intense grief or guilt

---

About This Chapter: This chapter includes text excerpted from "Suicide And PTSD," U.S. Department of Veterans Affairs (VA), October 1, 2015.

several months after the suicide, contact a mental health provider for help. Many people feel guilty about not having prevented the suicide. Be aware, though, that suicide is never your fault. Suicide is complex with many factors that contribute. It can also be difficult to cope when a loved one has made a suicide attempt.

What Does "Suicide Contagion" Mean, And What Can Be Done To Prevent It?

Suicide contagion is the exposure to suicide or suicidal behaviors within one's family, one's peer group, or through media reports of suicide and can result in an increase in suicide and suicidal behaviors. Direct and indirect exposure to suicidal behavior has been shown to precede an increase in suicidal behavior in persons at risk for suicide, especially in adolescents and young adults.

Following exposure to suicide or suicidal behaviors within one's family or peer group, suicide risk can be minimized by having family members, friends, peers, and colleagues of the victim evaluated by a mental health professional. Persons deemed at risk for suicide should then be referred for additional mental health services.

(Source: "What Does "Suicide Contagion" Mean, And What Can Be Done To Prevent It?" U.S. Department of Health and Human Services (HHS).)

Part Five
Preventing Suicide

Chapter 38
What Is Mental Health?

"Mental health" refers to your emotional, psychological, and social well-being. Your mental health affects how you think, feel, and act. It also helps determine how you handle stress, relate to others, and make choices.

Positive mental health allows you to:

- realize your full potential

- cope with the stresses of life

- work productively

- make meaningful contributions to your community

Positive mental health is important for all individuals at every stage of life.

Children's Mental Health

The term childhood mental disorder means all mental disorders that can be diagnosed and begin in childhood (for example, attention deficit hyperactivity disorder (ADHD), Tourette syndrome, behavior disorders, mood and anxiety disorders, autism spectrum disorders, substance use disorders, etc.). Mental disorders among children are described as serious changes in the ways children typically learn, behave, or handle their emotions. Symptoms usually start in early childhood, although some of the disorders may develop throughout the teenage years.

About This Chapter: Text in this chapter begins with excerpts from "Mental Health," AIDS.gov, U.S. Department of Health and Human Services (HHS), March 7, 2014; Text beginning with the heading "Children's Mental Health" is excerpted from "Children's Mental Health—New Report," Centers for Disease Control and Prevention (CDC), May 16, 2013. Reviewed January 2017.

The diagnosis is often made in the school years and sometimes earlier. However, some children with a mental disorder may not be recognized or diagnosed as having one.

Childhood mental disorders can be treated and managed. There are many evidence-based treatment options, so parents and doctors should work closely with everyone involved in the child's treatment—teachers, coaches, therapists, and other family members. Taking advantage of all the resources available will help parents, health professionals and educators guide the child towards success. Early diagnosis and appropriate services for children and their families can make a difference in the lives of children with mental disorders.

Early Warning Signs Of Mental Health Issues

Not sure if you or someone you know is living with mental health problems? Experiencing one or more of the following feelings or behaviors can be an early warning sign of a problem:

- eating or sleeping too much or too little
- pulling away from people and usual activities
- having low or no energy
- feeling numb or like nothing matters
- having unexplained aches and pains
- feeling helpless or hopeless
- smoking, drinking, or using drugs more than usual
- feeling unusually confused, forgetful, on edge, angry, upset, worried, or scared
- yelling or fighting with family and friends
- experiencing severe mood swings that cause problems in relationships
- having persistent thoughts and memories you can't get out of your head
- hearing voices or believing things that are not true
- thinking of harming yourself or others
- inability to perform daily tasks like taking care of your kids or getting to work or school

(Source: "What Is Mental Health," MentalHealth.gov, U.S. Department of Health and Human Services (HHS).)

An Important Public Health Issue

Mental health is important to overall health. Mental disorders are chronic health conditions that can continue through the lifespan. Without early diagnosis and treatment, children with mental disorders can have problems at home, in school, and in forming friendships.

This can also interfere with their healthy development, and these problems can continue into adulthood.

Children's mental disorders affect many children and families. Boys and girls of all ages, ethnic/racial backgrounds, and regions of the United States experience mental disorders. Based on the National Research Council and Institute of Medicine report (*Preventing Mental, Emotional, and Behavioral Disorders Among Young People: Progress and Possibilities*, 2009) that gathered findings from previous studies, it is estimated that 13–20 percent of children living in the United States (up to 1 out of 5 children) experience a mental disorder in a given year and an estimated $247 billion is spent each year on childhood mental disorders. Because of the impact on children, families, and communities, children's mental disorders are an important public health issue in the United States.

Public health surveillance—which is the collection and monitoring of information about health among the public over time—is a first step to better understand childhood mental disorders and promote children's mental health. Ongoing and systematic monitoring of mental health and mental disorders will help:

- increase understanding of the mental health needs of children

- inform research on factors that increase risk and promote prevention

- find out which programs are effective at preventing mental disorders and promoting children's mental health

- monitor if treatment and prevention efforts are effective

Who Is Affected?

The following are key findings from this report about mental disorders among children aged 3–17 years:

- Millions of American children live with depression, anxiety, ADHD, autism spectrum disorders, Tourette syndrome or a host of other mental health issues.

- ADHD was the most prevalent current diagnosis among children aged 3–17 years.

- The number of children with a mental disorder increased with age, with the exception of autism spectrum disorders, which was highest among 6 to 11 year old children.

- Boys were more likely than girls to have ADHD, behavioral or conduct problems, autism spectrum disorders, anxiety, Tourette syndrome, and cigarette dependence.

- Adolescent boys aged 12–17 years were more likely than girls to die by suicide.

- Adolescent girls were more likely than boys to have depression or an alcohol use disorder.

What You Can Do

Parents: You know your child best. Talk to your child's healthcare professional if you have concerns about the way your child behaves at home, in school, or with friends.

Youth: It is just as important to take care of your mental health as it is your physical health. If you are angry, worried or sad, don't be afraid to talk about your feelings and reach out to a trusted friend or adult.

Healthcare professionals: Early diagnosis and appropriate treatment based on updated guidelines is very important. There are resources available to help diagnose and treat children's mental disorders.

Teachers / School Administrators: Early identification is important, so that children can get the help they need. Work with families and healthcare professionals if you have concerns about the mental health of a child in your school.

Chapter 39
Coping With Stress

Feeling Stressed

Schoolwork, chores, dating dramas, fights with friends, and more—so many things can stress you out! But what exactly is stress, and how can you handle it?

What Is Stress?

Stress is what you feel when you react to pressure. The pressure can come from events in your life, from other people, or even from yourself. Things that cause stress are called stressors.

What Causes Stress?

Different people are stressed by different things. For example, you might get very stressed about a test, but your friend might feel fine. Your sister might think moving is terrifying, but you may think it's exciting. There are no right or wrong things to stress over.

Some things that might cause stress include:

- schoolwork

- changes in your body or weight

- problems with friends or other relationships

- being bullied

About This Chapter: Text under the heading "Feeling Stressed" is excerpted from "Feeling Stressed," girlshealth. gov, Office on Women's Health (OWH), January 7, 2015; Text under the heading "Stress And The Risk Of Suicide" is excerpted from "The Sorrow Of Suicide," *NIH News in Health*, National Institutes of Health (NIH), May 2012. Reviewed January 2017.

- living in a dangerous neighborhood

- peer pressure to dress or act a certain way, or to smoke, drink, or use drugs

- feeling like you don't fit in

- desire to please your parents or other important adults

- sick family member

- changing schools

- conflict at home

- taking on too many activities at once

Of course, other things may cause stress for you that are not listed above. Even fun things, like starring in the school play or starting to date, can get you stressed.

Some things that cause stress are the same things that cause grief. These include things like your parents getting divorced or the death of someone you love.

Is Stress Always Bad?

A little bit of stress can help you. During a sports competition, stress might push you to perform better, for example. Also, the stress of deadlines can get you to finish work on time.

A lot of stress or stress that lasts a long time can hurt you. It can cause problems for your physical and emotional health, like stomach aches, sleep problems, and trouble concentrating.

If your stress is getting to be too much, take steps to tackle it. Also, turn to a parent or another adult you trust for advice and support.

Don't try to lower your stress in unhealthy ways. Things like taking drugs, drinking, cutting back on your sleep, or eating a lot or very little will only cause more problems. Treat yourself with the respect you deserve.

What Are Signs Of Being Stressed Out?

Sometimes, stress just comes and goes. But if you are facing a lot of pressure or problems, you may start to feel like you're often too stressed out.

Signs that you are getting too stressed may include:

- feeling down or tired

- feeling angry or edgy

- feeling sad or worried

- having trouble concentrating

- having headaches or stomach aches

- having trouble sleeping

- laughing or crying for no reason

- wanting to be alone a lot

- having tense muscles

- not being able to see the positive side of a situation

- not enjoying activities that you used to enjoy

- feeling like you have too many things you have to do

Some of these signs can also be signs of depression, which needs treatment.

How Does My Body Act When Stressed?

Your body has a built-in response to stressors. Your palms may sweat, your mouth may get dry, and your stomach may twist. This is all normal! Of course, stress doesn't feel very good. When your body is hit by stress, try to calm it down. Taking some deep breaths can help. You also can try yoga, going for a walk, or some other physical activity.

Can Stress Lead To More Serious Problems?

Stress that's too much for you to handle may play a role in some serious problems. These problems include eating disorders, hurting yourself, depression, anxiety disorders, alcohol and drug abuse, smoking, and even suicide. If you are facing any of these problems, talk to an adult you trust right away! You also can get support by phone, text, chat, or email from a special helpline for teens.

What Are Ways To Handle Stress?

Put Your Body In Motion

Physical activity is a great way to beat stress. It can clear your head and lift your spirits. Physical activity increases endorphins, which are natural "feel-good" chemicals in the body. You may like games of football, tennis, or basketball, or you may prefer walks with family and friends. Whatever you choose, get up, get out, and get moving!

Fuel Up

When you take a car for a long drive, you fill up the gas tank first. You also need to fuel your body each day.

Balanced nutrition gives you the energy you need to handle hectic days. Don't be fooled by the jolt of energy you get from sodas and sugary snacks. The boost is short, and when it wears off, you may feel even more tired. Start the day with a healthy breakfast. If you don't feel like eating when you wake up, grab a healthy snack like a banana, string cheese, or nuts so you can fuel up on the go.

LOL!

Laughter may not be the best medicine, but it sure can help. Lots of laughing can help your body make natural "feel-good" chemicals called endorphins. And the good feeling can last after the giggling stops. So, beat stress with a funny movie, cartoons, or jokes.

We all do things we think are pretty silly or stupid at times. When you do, try not to get mad at yourself. Instead, see if you can find the funny in what you did.

Have Fun With Friends

Being with people you like is a good way to ditch your stress. Get a group together to watch a movie, shoot some hoops, listen to music—or just hang out and talk. Friends can help you remember the brighter side of life.

Spill To Someone You Trust

Instead of keeping your feelings bottled up, talk to someone you trust about what's bothering you. It could be a friend, a parent, a teacher, or a friend's parent. The person may have some great advice or a different way to look at things. Plus, just getting support can feel good. Remember, you don't have to handle stress alone!

Take Time To Chill

Pick a comfy spot to sit and read, daydream, or take a nap. Listen to your favorite music. Work on a relaxing project like doing a puzzle or making jewelry.

Stress can sometimes make you feel like a rubber band pulled tight. If this happens, take a few deep breaths. If you're in the middle of an impossible homework problem, take a break! Taking time to relax after (and sometimes during) a hectic day can make a big difference.

Catch Some ZZZ's

Being stressed out can affect your sleep, which can make you feel cranky or fuzzy-headed. Being tired can mess up schoolwork, sports, friendships, and more. All that can add to your stress!

Sleep is a big deal for teens. Because your body and mind are changing, you need more sleep to recharge for the next day. Most teens should aim for a little more than 9 hours of sleep each night. Get tips for better sleep.

Keep A Journal

Having a hard day? You can write about what's going on and how you feel. Writing is a great way to get things off your chest. You also can write a plan for how to handle problems and responsibilities. Then, you might go back and reread what you wrote a couple of weeks later to see how you got through a tough time. You can create your own journal.

Get It Together

Feeling overwhelmed or forgetful? Being unprepared for school, practice, or other activities can make for a very stressful day. Having a plan and getting organized can really help. You can learn ways to manage your time well.

Lend A Hand

Helping someone can help you feel capable and strong. And it can remind you that everyone faces some kind of challenge at some point. Helping others also is a great way to find out about talents you never knew you had!

You can help in simple ways, like smiling at someone who looks sad or helping an older neighbor with packages. If you want to join a volunteer group, try contacting a local recreation center or after-school program.

Stress And The Risk Of Suicide

Suicide is the 10th leading cause of death nationwide, and it's the 3rd leading cause of death among adolescents.

It cuts a life short, and it devastates the family, friends and loved ones left behind. Those who survive a suicide attempt might end up with severe disability or other injuries. The children of people who die by suicide are more likely to later die by suicide themselves. With such extreme consequences, why would anyone make the dire decision to choose death over life?

People of all genders, ages and ethnicities are at risk for suicide. Women are more likely than men to attempt suicide, but men are more likely to die by suicide. That's because men often choose deadlier methods, such as firearms or suffocation.

Suicide risk is also higher among people who have certain mental disorders, including schizophrenia and bipolar disorder. Depression affects more than half of those who die by suicide. Other risk factors include a prior suicide attempt, a family history of suicide, substance abuse, or having guns or other firearms in the home.

"Stress and trauma certainly play a big role in suicide, especially early life stress," says Dr. Douglas Meinecke, an National Institutes of Health (NIH) scientist who studies the molecular details of mental disorders. Several research teams have found evidence that traumatic childhood experiences—such as abuse or violence—can "tag" certain genes in the brain. These tags, called epigenetic markers, are actually molecules that attach to genes. They can have a lasting effect on whether the genes are turned off or on.

Some NIH-funded studies have shown that suicide victims who were abused as children have unique epigenetic markers on certain genes. These markers were not found in suicide victims with no history of childhood abuse or in people who died in accidents. More research into how stress affects genes and suicide risk might offer new chances for early intervention.

Current approaches to treating or preventing suicide generally aim to relieve the accompanying mental condition or other risk factors. "If you focus on making people who have mental disorders as well as they can be, managing life as well as they can or reducing their suicidal thoughts, you can greatly reduce suicide overall," says Meinecke.

Medications—such as antidepressants and antipsychotics—can help. Psychotherapy, or "talk therapy," can also be effective. One type, called cognitive behavioral therapy (CBT), can help people learn new ways to deal with stressful situations by training them to consider alternative actions when thoughts of suicide arise.

One of the most effective tools for preventing suicide is to know the warning signs and take quick action to get the person into treatment. "One of the biggest indicators of suicide risk is when somebody begins talking about suicide," says Dr. David Brent, a psychiatrist at the University of Pittsburgh who studies suicide in families. "We used to think that talking about suicide meant you weren't going to do it, but it's really the opposite. Other warning signs include withdrawal from usual activities, a change in mood or a change in sleep patterns."

Never ignore someone's talk of suicide. You can ask directly if the person has ever thought of harming himself or herself. Most people will answer honestly, and the question itself won't push a person to attempt suicide.

5 Things You Should Know About Stress

1. Stress affects everyone.
2. Not all stress is bad.
3. Long-term stress can harm your health.
4. There are ways to manage stress.
5. If you're overwhelmed by stress, ask for help from a health professional.

(Source: "5 Things You Should Know About Stress," National Institute of Mental Health (NIMH).)

Chapter 40
Sleep Is Vital To Your Well-Being

Lack Of Sleep And The Risk Of Suicide

After a good night's sleep, we feel rested, refreshed, and ready to take on the day. But after a poor night's sleep, we may face the day tired, fatigued, irritable, and with less ability to focus. An estimated 70 million Americans are affected by lack of sleep and other sleeping disorders, making insufficient sleep a public health epidemic. Chronic lack of sleep has also been associated with certain physical and mental health disorders, such as diabetes, obesity, depression, anxiety, and as a growing body of evidence suggests, suicidal behavior.

Sleep And Its Vitality

Sleep plays a vital role in good health and well-being throughout your life. Getting enough quality sleep at the right times can help protect your mental health, physical health, quality of life, and safety.

The way you feel while you're awake depends in part on what happens while you're sleeping. During sleep, your body is working to support healthy brain function and maintain your physical health. In children and teens, sleep also helps support growth and development.

About This Chapter: Text under the heading "Lack Of Sleep And The Risk Of Suicide" is excerpted from "Sleep, Suicide And Research For Veterans" Mental Illness Research, Education and Clinical Center (MIRECC), U.S. Department of Veterans Affairs (VA), August 2015. Text beginning with the heading "Sleep And Its Vitality" is excerpted from "Why Is Sleep Important?" National Heart, Lung, and Blood Institute (NHLBI), February 22, 2012. Reviewed January 2017; Text under the heading "Most U.S. Middle And High Schools Start The School Day Too Early" is excerpted from "Most U.S. Middle And High Schools Start The School Day Too Early," Centers for Disease Control and Prevention (CDC), August 6, 2015; Text under the heading "Teen Sleep Habits" is excerpted from "Teen Sleep Habits," Centers for Disease Control and Prevention (CDC), October 13, 2011. Reviewed January 2017.

The damage from sleep deficiency can occur in an instant (such as a car crash), or it can harm you over time. For example, ongoing sleep deficiency can raise your risk for some chronic health problems. It also can affect how well you think, react, work, learn, and get along with others.

The Connection Between Suicide And Sleep Problems

It may not seem like there would be a connection but if you think about how important sleep is to humans, it begins to make a lot of sense. Sleep is very important because it is rejuvenating, it's refreshing, and it helps us function optimally during the day. Conversely, if we're not sleeping well, we're not performing optimally; we're a little tired, we're a little irritable, we're a little frustrated, and if that continues over time it becomes an additional stressor on our system. We don't know precisely why there is a connection between sleep and suicidal thoughts and attempts and even death, but there is a connection. One thought is simply that poor sleep is an additional stressor, on top of many other stressors, that a person may have to deal with in their life. It might be the difference between having a very fleeting suicidal thought every once in a while, and having more chronic, persistent suicidal thoughts. It might be the difference between having suicidal thoughts and acting on those thoughts.

Healthy Brain Function And Emotional Well-Being

Sleep helps your brain work properly. While you're sleeping, your brain is preparing for the next day. It's forming new pathways to help you learn and remember information.

Studies show that a good night's sleep improves learning. Whether you're learning math, how to play the piano, how to perfect your golf swing, or how to drive a car, sleep helps enhance your learning and problem-solving skills. Sleep also helps you pay attention, make decisions, and be creative.

Studies also show that sleep deficiency alters activity in some parts of the brain. If you're sleep deficient, you may have trouble making decisions, solving problems, controlling your emotions and behavior, and coping with change. Sleep deficiency also has been linked to depression, suicide, and risk-taking behavior.

Children and teens who are sleep deficient may have problems getting along with others. They may feel angry and impulsive, have mood swings, feel sad or depressed, or lack motivation. They also may have problems paying attention, and they may get lower grades and feel stressed.

Physical Health

Sleep plays an important role in your physical health. For example, sleep is involved in healing and repair of your heart and blood vessels. Ongoing sleep deficiency is linked to an increased risk of heart disease, kidney disease, high blood pressure, diabetes, and stroke.

Sleep deficiency also increases the risk of obesity. For example, one study of teenagers showed that with each hour of sleep lost, the odds of becoming obese went up. Sleep deficiency increases the risk of obesity in other age groups as well.

Sleep helps maintain a healthy balance of the hormones that make you feel hungry (ghrelin) or full (leptin). When you don't get enough sleep, your level of ghrelin goes up and your level of leptin goes down. This makes you feel hungrier than when you're well-rested.

Sleep also affects how your body reacts to insulin, the hormone that controls your blood glucose (sugar) level. Sleep deficiency results in a higher than normal blood sugar level, which may increase your risk for diabetes.

Sleep also supports healthy growth and development. Deep sleep triggers the body to release the hormone that promotes normal growth in children and teens. This hormone also boosts muscle mass and helps repair cells and tissues in children, teens, and adults. Sleep also plays a role in puberty and fertility.

Your immune system relies on sleep to stay healthy. This system defends your body against foreign or harmful substances. Ongoing sleep deficiency can change the way in which your immune system responds. For example, if you're sleep deficient, you may have trouble fighting common infections.

Daytime Performance And Safety

Getting enough quality sleep at the right times helps you function well throughout the day. People who are sleep deficient are less productive at work and school. They take longer to finish tasks, have a slower reaction time, and make more mistakes.

After several nights of losing sleep—even a loss of just 1–2 hours per night—your ability to function suffers as if you haven't slept at all for a day or two.

Lack of sleep also may lead to microsleep. Microsleep refers to brief moments of sleep that occur when you're normally awake.

You can't control microsleep, and you might not be aware of it. For example, have you ever driven somewhere and then not remembered part of the trip? If so, you may have experienced microsleep.

Even if you're not driving, microsleep can affect how you function. If you're listening to a lecture, for example, you might miss some of the information or feel like you don't understand the point. In reality, though, you may have slept through part of the lecture and not been aware of it.

Some people aren't aware of the risks of sleep deficiency. In fact, they may not even realize that they're sleep deficient. Even with limited or poor-quality sleep, they may still think that they can function well.

For example, drowsy drivers may feel capable of driving. Yet, studies show that sleep deficiency harms your driving ability as much as, or more than, being drunk. It's estimated that driver sleepiness is a factor in about 100,000 car accidents each year, resulting in about 1,500 deaths.

Drivers aren't the only ones affected by sleep deficiency. It can affect people in all lines of work, including healthcare workers, pilots, students, lawyers, mechanics, and assembly line workers.

As a result, sleep deficiency is not only harmful on a personal level, but it also can cause large-scale damage. For example, sleep deficiency has played a role in human errors linked to tragic accidents, such as nuclear reactor meltdowns, grounding of large ships, and aviation accidents.

Most U.S. Middle And High Schools Start The School Day Too Early

Students need adequate sleep for their health, safety, and academic success.

Fewer than 1 in 5 middle and high schools in the United States began the school day at the recommended 8:30 AM start time or later during the 2011–2012 school year, according to data published in the Centers for Disease Control and Prevention's (CDC) Morbidity and Mortality Weekly Report (MMWR). Too-early start times can keep students from getting the sleep they need for health, safety, and academic success, according to the American Academy of Pediatrics.

CDC and U.S. Department of Education (ED) researchers reviewed data from the 2011–2012 Schools and Staffing Survey of nearly 40,000 public middle, high, and combined schools to determine school start times.

Schools that have a start time of 8:30 AM or later allow adolescent students the opportunity to get the recommended amount of sleep on school nights: about 8.5 to 9.5 hours. Insufficient sleep is common among high school students and is associated with several health risks such as being overweight, drinking alcohol, smoking tobacco, and using drugs—as well as poor academic performance. The proportion of high school students who fail to get sufficient sleep (2 out of 3) has remained steady since 2007, according to the 2013 Youth Risk Behavior Surveillance Report.

"Getting enough sleep is important for students' health, safety, and academic performance," said Anne Wheaton, Ph.D., lead author and epidemiologist in CDC's Division of Population Health. "Early school start times, however, are preventing many adolescents from getting the sleep they need."

In 2014, the American Academy of Pediatrics (AAP) issued a policy statement urging middle and high schools to modify start times to no earlier than 8:30 AM to aid students in getting sufficient sleep to improve their overall health. School start time policies are not determined at the federal or state level, but at the district or individual school level. Future studies may determine whether this recommendation results in later school start times.

Delayed school start times do not replace the need for other interventions that can improve sleep among adolescents. Parents can help their children practice good sleep habits. For example, a consistent bedtime and rise time, including on weekends, is recommended for everyone, including children, adolescents, and adults. Healthcare providers who treat adolescents should educate teens and parents about the importance of adequate sleep in maintaining health and well-being.

Teen Sleep Habits

Almost 70 percent of high school students are not getting the recommended hours of sleep on school nights, according to a study by the CDC. Researchers found insufficient sleep (<8 hours on an average school night) to be associated with a number of unhealthy activities, such as:

- drinking soda or pop 1 or more times per day (not including diet soda or diet pop)
- not participating in 60 minutes of physical activity on 5 or more of the past 7 days
- using computers 3 or more hours each day
- being in a physical fight 1 or more times
- cigarette use

- alcohol use

- marijuana use

- current sexual activity

- feeling sad or hopeless

- seriously considering attempting suicide

Adolescents not getting sufficient sleep each night may be due to changes in the sleep/wake cycle as well as everyday activities, such as employment, recreational activities, academic pressures, early school start times, and access to technology.

> The National Sleep Foundation recommends that teenagers receive between 8.5 hours and 9.25 hours each night.

The following sleep health tips are recommended by the National Sleep Foundation:

- Go to bed at the same time each night and rise at the same time each morning.

- Make sure your bedroom is a quiet, dark, and relaxing environment, which is neither too hot or too cold.

- Make sure your bed is comfortable and use it only for sleeping and not for other activities, such as reading, watching TV, or listening to music. Remove all TVs, computers, and other "gadgets" from the bedroom.

- Avoid large meals a few hours before bedtime.

If your sleep problems persist or if they interfere with how you feel or function during the day, you should seek the assistance of a physician or other health professional. Before visiting your physician, consider keeping a diary of your sleep habits for about ten days to discuss at the visit.

Include the following in your sleep diary, when you:

- go to bed

- go to sleep

- wake up

- get out of bed

- take naps

- exercise

- consume alcohol and how much

- consume caffeinated beverages and how much

Chapter 41
Body Image And Self-Esteem

Having Body Image Issues

Do you wish you could lose weight, get taller, or develop faster? It's pretty common to worry a little about how your body looks, especially when it's changing. You can learn about body image and ways to take control of yours.

What Is Body Image?

Body image is how you think and feel about your body. It includes whether you think you look good to other people.

Body image is affected by a lot of things, including messages you get from your friends, family, and the world around you. Images we see in the media definitely affect our body image even though a lot of media images are changed or aren't realistic.

Why does body image matter? Your body image can affect how you feel about yourself overall. For example, if you are unhappy with your looks, your self-esteem may start to go down. Sometimes, having body image issues or low self-esteem may lead to depression, eating disorders, or obesity.

About This Chapter: Text under the heading "Having Body Image Issues" is excerpted from "Having Body Image Issues," girlshealth.gov, Office on Women's Health (OWH), January 7, 2015; Text under the heading "Ways To Build Self-Esteem" is excerpted from "Ways To Build Self-Esteem," girlshealth.gov, Office on Women's Health (OWH), February 16, 2011. Reviewed January 2017.

How Can I Deal With Body Image Issues?

Everyone has something they would like to change about their bodies. But you'll be happier if you focus on the things you like about your body—and your whole self. Need some help? Check out some tips:

- **List your great traits.** If you start to criticize your body, tell yourself to stop. Instead, think about what you like about yourself, both inside and out.

- **Know your power.** Hey, your body is not just a place to hang your clothes! It can do some truly amazing things. Focus on how strong and healthy your body can be.

- **Treat your body well.** Eat right, sleep tight, and get moving. You'll look and feel your best—and you'll be pretty proud of yourself too.

- **Give your body a treat.** Take a nice bubble bath, do some stretching, or just curl up on a comfy couch. Do something soothing.

- **Mind your media.** Try not to let models and actresses affect how you think you should look. They get lots of help from makeup artists, personal trainers, and photo fixers. And advertisers often use a focus on thinness to get people to buy stuff. Don't let them mess with your mind!

- **Let yourself shine.** A lot of how we look comes from how we carry ourselves. Feeling proud, walking tall, and smiling big can boost your beauty—and your mood.

- **Find fabulous friends.** Your best bet is to hang out with people who accept you for you! And work with your friends to support each other.

If you can't seem to accept how you look, talk to an adult you trust. You can get help feeling better about your body.

Stressing About Body Changes

During puberty and your teen years, your body changes a lot. All those changes can be hard to handle. They might make you worry about what other people think of how you look and about whether your body is normal. If you have these kinds of concerns, you are not alone.

Here are some common thoughts about changing bodies.

- Why am I taller than most of the boys my age?

- Why haven't I grown?

- Am I too skinny?

- Am I too fat?

- Will others like me now that I am changing?

- Are my breasts too small?

- Are my breasts too large?

- Why do I have acne?

- Do my clothes look right on my body?

- Are my hips getting bigger?

If you are stressed about your body, you may feel better if you understand why you are changing so fast—or not changing as fast as your friends.

During puberty, you get taller and see other changes in your body, such as wider hips and thighs. Your body will also start to have more fat compared to muscle than before. Each young woman changes at her own pace, and all of these changes are normal.

What Are Serious Body Image Problems?

If how your body looks bothers you a lot and you can't stop thinking about it, you could have body dysmorphic disorder, or BDD.

People with BDD think they look ugly even if they have a small flaw or none at all. They may spend many hours a day looking at flaws and trying to hide them. They also may ask friends to reassure them about their looks or want to have a lot of cosmetic surgery. If you or a friend may have BDD, talk to an adult you trust, such as a parent or guardian, school counselor, teacher, doctor, or nurse. BDD is an illness, and you can get help.

> Having a negative body image like this isn't just an attitude problem. It can take a toll on your mental and physical health. If excessive thoughts about your body cause great distress or interfere with your daily life, you may have a body image disorder, also known as body dysmorphic disorder (BDD). Because of their imagined flaws, many people with BDD avoid going out in public or shun friends and family. About three-quarters have had major depression, and about 1 in 4 attempt suicide.
>
> *(Source: "How You See Yourself," NIH News in Health, National Institutes of Health (NIH).)*

Ways To Build Self-Esteem

Having healthy or high self-esteem means that you feel good about yourself and are proud of what you can do. Having high self-esteem can help you to think positively, deal better with stress, and boost your drive to work hard. Having high self-esteem can also make it easier to try new things. Before you try something new, you think, "I can do this," and not, "This is too hard. I'll never be able to do this."

If you have an illness or disability, how does it affect your self-esteem? Do you find your self-esteem is affected by how you think others see you? Do people put you down or bully you? This can put your self-esteem at risk. If you need a self-esteem boost, take these steps:

- **Ask yourself what you are really good at and enjoy doing.** Everyone is good at something. When you're feeling bad about yourself, just think, "I'm good at art" (or computers or playing an instrument or whatever you're good at). You might make a list of your great traits and talents, too. And remember that it's okay not to be great at everything.

- **Push yourself to try new things.** If you try something new and fail, that's okay. Everyone fails sometime. Try to figure out what went wrong, so you can try again in a new way. Keep trying, and don't give up. In time, you'll figure out how to succeed.

- **Always give your best effort, and take pride in your effort.** When you accomplish a goal, celebrate over a family meal or treat yourself to a fun outing.

- **If you need help, ask for it.** Talking to a parent, teacher, or friend can help you come up with different ways to solve a problem. This is called brainstorming. Make a list of your possible solutions. Put the ones that you think will work the best at the top. Then rehearse them ahead of time so that you'll know exactly what you're going to do or say when the problem comes up. If your first plan doesn't work, then go on to Plan B. If Plan B doesn't work, go on to Plan C, and so on.

- **Join a support group.** Finding out how other kids deal with illnesses or disabilities can help you cope. Ask your doctor, teachers, or parents for help finding a support group in your community or online.

- **Volunteer to do something at school or in your community.** For instance, you could tutor a younger child or take care of the plants in the community center lobby. You might also volunteer to do some chores at home.

- **Look for ways to take more control over your life.** For instance, every student who has needs related to an illness or disability in school must have an Individualized Education

Plan, or IEP. Your IEP describes your goals during the school year and any support that you'll need to help achieve those goals. Get involved with the development of your IEP. Attend any IEP meetings. Tell your parents, teachers, and others involved in your IEP what you think your goals at school should be and what would help you achieve them. It's your education, and you get a say in what happens!

- **Speak up for yourself.** This can be difficult if you're shy. But it can get easier with practice. Learn to communicate your needs and don't hesitate to ask for something.

- **Work on trying to feel good about how you look.** Everyone has some things they like and don't like about their bodies. It pays to focus on the positives since your body image, or how you feel about your looks, can affect your self-esteem. And remember that real beauty comes from the inside! If you like makeup and clothes, ask for help dealing with any obstacles your illness or disability might present.

- **If you still find that you are not feeling good about yourself, talk to your parents, a school counselor, or your doctor because you may be at risk for depression.** You can also ask the school nurse if your school offers counseling for help through tough times.

> If you don't have a body image disorder, improving your attitude about your body might just be a matter of accepting that healthy bodies come in many shapes and sizes. We all want to look good, but you should never sacrifice your health to try to achieve a "perfect" body.
>
> *(Source: "How You See Yourself," NIH News in Health, National Institutes of Health (NIH).)*

Chapter 42

Helping A Depressed Person

Depression is not the same as sadness. Everyone feels sad sometimes. That's normal. Depression also involves things like feeling hopeless and having very little energy.

Depression can feel absolutely awful. It can kill your energy, steal your joy, and ruin your friendships. Sometimes depression is mild and your life doesn't feel completely changed. Other times, depression is very strong and you might feel like everything is hopeless. But treatment for depression works well. If you think you have depression, get help. You can feel better!

Depression in teens is pretty common. In fact, around 2 million U.S. teens had major depression at some point, according to a recent survey. Learning about depression can help you and others.

Girls And Depression
Before puberty, boys and girls face equal chances of getting some form of depression. But between the ages of 12 and 17, girls are about three times as likely as boys to have major depression.

Could I Have Depression?

Everybody feels down sometimes. Usually, we get over it quickly, like in a couple of days. But depression can stick around for weeks or months.

About This Chapter: This chapter includes text excerpted from "Depression," girlshealth.gov, Office on Women's Health (OWH), January 7, 2015.

You could have depression and not know it. If you have depression, you might feel really bad about yourself or about your life but not know why. Keep reading to learn signs that you may have depression.

If you have some of the following issues and they get in the way of your day-to-day life, get help.

- Sadness or crying that you can't explain

- Big changes in the way you eat, such as overeating or not eating

- Being crabby, irritable, angry, or restless

- Being worried or nervous

- Feeling negative, guilty, or worthless

- Sleep changes, such as sleeping more or having trouble sleeping

- Trouble focusing or making decisions

- Not being able to enjoy the things you usually enjoy

- Not wanting to spend time with your friends

- Feeling tired most of the time or not having the energy to do things

- Having aches or pains that don't go away

- Thinking about death or suicide

It's important to get help if you think you may have depression. Treatment can help you feel so much better. If your depression doesn't get treated, it can get worse. Also, the sooner you get treatment, the better it may work.

People who have depression may try to lessen their pain in unhealthy ways. A person who is depressed may try cutting herself to turn the pain into something physical. She might look for escape by trying drugs or alcohol or eating a lot of food. She might even try drinking a lot of energy drinks for a boost. None of these will make depression go away. In fact, all of these can make problems worse and create new problems. If you have depression, talk to people who care about you, and get help from a mental health professional.

Teens also can have other mental health conditions. These might come alone or together with depression.

Getting Help For Depression

Treatment for depression usually works really well. Treatment can include medicine and talk therapy. You can learn more about getting help through medicine and about therapy.

If you think you may need treatment for depression, you can start by talking to your parents or guardians.

Helping Someone Who Is Depressed

Lots of young people feel sad or stressed at times. But if you know someone who has been down for weeks, that person may be dealing with depression. Don't be afraid to ask if that person is having trouble. Talking about depression does not make it worse, but ignoring it can.

Here are some tips for helping someone who may be depressed:

- **Encourage the person to get help.** Many teens don't look for the help they need. That's too bad, because treatment can work well.

- **Talk with a trusted adult.** A depressed person may feel too drained or hopeless to get help. You are doing the person a big favor by talking to a caring adult for them.

- **Be patient.** Depression is a real illness. Someone who has it can't just decide to be in a better mood.

- **Talk and listen.** Offer support and understanding. Pay attention when the other person wants to talk.

- **Never shoot down the other person's feelings.** Arguing won't help. You can't convince a depressed person that their life is okay. You can say how you see things, though. Just remember to be gentle.

- **Offer hope.** Remind the person that with time and treatment, depression definitely can get better.

- **Invite the person out.** Suggest something simple, like a walk. Keep trying if the person says no, but don't be pushy.

- **Never ignore comments about suicide.** Talk to the person's parent or guardian or to a teacher, school counselor, school nurse, or doctor.

5 Action Steps For Helping Someone In Emotional Pain

- **Ask:** "Are you thinking about killing yourself?" It's not an easy question but studies show that asking at-risk individuals if they are suicidal does not increase suicides or suicidal thoughts.

- **Keep them safe:** Reducing a suicidal person's access to highly lethal items or places is an important part of suicide prevention. While this is not always easy, asking if the at-risk person has a plan and removing or disabling the lethal means can make a difference.

- **Be there:** Listen carefully and learn what the individual is thinking and feeling. Findings suggest acknowledging and talking about suicide may in fact reduce rather than increase suicidal thoughts.

- **Help them connect:** Save the National Suicide Prevention Lifeline's number in your phone so it's there when you need it: 800-273-TALK (800-273-8255). You can also help make a connection with a trusted individual like a family member, friend, spiritual advisor, or mental health professional.

- **Stay connected:** Staying in touch after a crisis or after being discharged from care can make a difference. Studies have shown the number of suicide deaths goes down when someone follows up with the at-risk person.

Chapter 43
Helping A Suicidal Person

How To Talk About Suicide

It may not be easy to talk about suicide or respond to someone who brings the topic up in conversation. Across almost all cultures, and especially in places where rates are higher than the general population, the subject of suicide carries with it the stigmas of depression and death, and the fear that just talking about it will make it happen. However, talking about suicide and listening to those who share suicidal thoughts or behaviors is an important tool that may be used not only to prevent suicide, but also to help those who have lost hope heal.

Warning signs and risk factors often provide signals that someone may be considering suicide. Warning signs are clues which can be subtle or obvious indications that someone may be thinking of ending their life. Risk factors are circumstances that may increase one's susceptibility to thoughts of suicide. If you see any warning signs and recognize any risk factors in someone, starting the conversation may save their life.

Suicide warning signs may include: withdrawal from friends and family, talking about or preoccupation with death, expression of hopelessness or worthlessness, loss of interest in favorite activities, giving away needed or favorite possessions, and/or making arrangements to put affairs in order.

About This Chapter: This chapter includes text excerpted from "How To Talk About Suicide," Indian Health Service (IHS), U.S. Department of Health and Human Services (HHS), July 8, 2014.

Warning Signs Of Suicide

If someone you know is showing one or more of the following behaviors, he or she may be thinking about suicide. Don't ignore these warning signs. Get help immediately.

- Talking about wanting to die or to kill oneself
- Looking for a way to kill oneself
- Talking about feeling hopeless or having no reason to live
- Talking about feeling trapped or in unbearable pain
- Talking about being a burden to others
- Increasing the use of alcohol or drugs
- Acting anxious or agitated; behaving recklessly
- Sleeping too little or too much
- Withdrawing or feeling isolated
- Showing rage or talking about seeking revenge
- Displaying extreme mood swings

Get Help

If you or someone you know needs help, call the National Suicide Prevention Lifeline. Trained crisis workers are available to talk 24 hours a day, 7 days a week.

If you think someone is in immediate danger, do not leave him or her alone—stay there and call 911.

(Source: "Suicidal Behavior," MentalHealth.gov, U.S. Department of Health and Human Services (HHS).)

Begin The Conversation

Before talking with someone you are concerned about, be sure to have suicide crisis resources available, including the National Suicide Prevention Lifeline number, 800–273–TALK (800–273–8255), and numbers and addresses of local crisis lines or treatment centers. Mention what signs prompted you to ask about how they are feeling. Mention the words used or behavior displayed that you or others have noticed in the person. This makes it more difficult for them to deny that something may be wrong. Say:

"I've noticed that you've mentioned feeling (hopeless, depressed, useless, like a burden, etc.) lately"

or

"You haven't been spending time with your friends and have been sleeping a lot lately"

Next, ask directly about suicide. Talking about suicide does NOT put the idea in someone's head and often provides some relief for that person since it gives them a chance to open up. Asking directly and using the word "suicide" establishes that you and the at-risk person are talking about the same thing and lets them know you are not afraid to talk about it:

"Sometimes when people feel that way, they think about suicide. Are you thinking about suicide?"

or

"Are you thinking about ending your life?"

If the answer is "yes" to your direct question, remain calm, and don't leave the person alone until you get help. Listen to the reasons the person gives for considering suicide as an option. Affirm that you realize what they are considering, but bring up that they may have felt differently before (which suggests that they may feel different again), and emphasize that living is an option for them:

"I can imagine how tough this must be for you. I know you say you're unsure if you want to live right now. But have you always felt like you wanted to die? It's possible you won't feel this way forever." Let the person know you care, that you take their situation seriously, that you are genuinely concerned, and will do all you can in your effort to support them:

"I'm deeply concerned about you and I want you to know that help is available to get you through this. I can help you."

Assess Risk

After you have established that they are considering suicide, ask the person if they have access to any lethal means (medications, weapons such as knives or guns, etc.) Say:

"Do you have any weapons, drugs, or prescription medications here?"

If the answer is yes, work to remove these items from the person's premises. You may need someone else—a friend, family member or even law enforcement—to assist with this task.

Develop A Safety Plan

Create a plan for keeping the person safe until you can get help. Ask the person what things (such as being in a certain place or having certain people around) will help keep them safe until they can meet or speak with a professional.

If it is an issue, ask the person if they will refrain from using alcohol and other drugs, or, if they can't or won't refrain, ask that they have someone who can monitor any use. Alcohol and drug use will lower inhibitions, change mood, cloud judgment, and may encourage a suicide attempt, and must be avoided, or at least watched closely:

"Will you promise you won't use alcohol or drugs, or at least have someone with you if you do, until we can get help?"

Get a verbal commitment that the person will not act upon thoughts of suicide until they have met with a professional:

"Please promise me that you will not harm yourself or act on any thoughts of suicide until you meet with a professional."

Get Help

Share the resources you have gathered with the person. Be willing to make the call, or to sit in on the call, to the National Suicide Prevention Lifeline at 800–273–TALK (800–273–8255). The toll-free confidential Lifeline is available 24 hours a day, seven days a week. Say to the person:

"You might not feel like going to talk to a counselor, but there's a number we can call to talk to somebody right now. Maybe they can help if we call?"

Let them know that you are willing to go with them to see a professional when they are ready. If you feel the situation is critical, take the person to a nearby Emergency Room or walk-in psychiatric crisis clinic if they are willing to go. If not, call 911. Do not put yourself in danger; if at any time during the process you are concerned about your own safety, or that the person may harm others, call 911.

Things Not To Say

Do not say *"You're not thinking about killing yourself, are you?"* Don't ask the person about suicide in a way that seems like you want to hear the answer "no." A "no" answer just gives the person the opportunity to shut down the conversation, limits your ability to gain the person's trust, and can end your chances of helping them.

Also, even if you are feeling upset and hurt, do not display anger, tell the person to do it, or tell them that you don't care, as these are the most dangerous things you can say. A suicidal person may be looking for any confirmation that they are unwanted, a burden, or will not be missed, and negative words may push them to act.

And never promise secrecy. The person may say that they don't want you to tell anyone that they are suicidal. You may be concerned that they will be angry with you if you tell others, but when a life is at risk, it is more important to ensure their safety. Instead, tell them you care about them too much and that you will help them get the assistance they need.

270

Chapter 44
Preventing Suicide Contagion

Suicide Contagion

There is some evidence that after a young person dies by suicide, other youth may attempt the same thing. This may lead to "suicide clusters"—an unexpectedly high number of suicides that occur close together in time or space. But these tragedies are preventable.

Understanding Suicide Clusters

Suicide is the second leading cause of death among college students, with an estimated 1,500 deaths each year. Because college suicides aren't officially tracked at the national or state level it's hard to know beyond anecdotal evidence how often clusters occur.

What's better known are the mechanisms behind suicide clusters—the process by which direct or indirect knowledge of a suicide facilitates subsequent suicides. One key factor is emotional suggestibility, noting people's tendency to identify with others, mimic their behavior, or even confuse other people's emotions as their own. For students who have already contemplated suicide, she said, a peer's suicide can "tip the balance" toward engaging in suicidal behavior themselves.

College students are especially vulnerable to suicide clusters since they're often away from their families for the first time and much more involved with peers. Plus, the part of the brain that helps control impulsiveness hasn't fully developed yet.

About This Chapter: Text under the heading "Suicide Contagion" is excerpted from "Suicide Cluster Prevention On Campus," Substance Abuse and Mental Health Services Administration (SAMHSA), December 3, 2015; Text under the heading "SAMHSA's Recommendations For Reporting On Suicide" is excerpted from "Recommendations For Reporting On Suicide," Substance Abuse and Mental Health Services Administration (SAMHSA), May 2011. Reviewed January 2017.

As a result, research shows a significant association between a peer's suicide and subsequent deaths. If someone in a peer group has attempted suicide or died by suicide, there's a 3 to 11 fold increase in the odds that a friend will actually attempt suicide.

Media coverage also has an impact—both positive and negative. When the media focuses on coping strategies—like being active, reaching out for support, and volunteering—rather than suicide, suicide rates decrease.

For this reason, Substance Abuse and Mental Health Services Administration (SAMHSA), together with several other organizations, developed a guide, Recommendations for Reporting on Suicide. The guide equips media with practical recommendations for covering suicide in ways that can change public perceptions and correct myths. It also offers tips to avoid misinformation and lists the warning signs of suicide.

Sharing The News

On the flip side, media messages can increase vulnerable people's risk and undermine prevention efforts.

Pictures or detailed descriptions of how and where a person died can encourage imitation and serve as a how-to guide. Another common mistake is oversimplifying the causes of suicide, attributing it to single factors like break-ups or bullying. Romanticizing suicide or portraying it as common may also feed into a false perception for someone who may be struggling with suicidal feelings.

Language use matters too. "Epidemic" suggests the problem is too big to solve, for instance, while "unsuccessful" or "failed attempt" imply that success equals suicide.

Several strategies can help campus administrators communicate safely and effectively:

- **Be prepared.** Make a plan before you need it. Identify who will share news with the campus community and how that person will communicate. Create customizable templates, drawing on the sample announcement letter in the Higher Education Mental Health Alliance's "Postvention: A Guide for Response to Suicide on College Campuses" (see: hemha.org/postvention_guide.pdf). (Decide what to do about memorial services. The plan should also include social media. To prevent the spread of rumors, post information about resources and monitor postings for unsafe content or cries for help.)

- **Focus on the positive.** The vast majority of people who face adversity or who live with mental illness don't die by suicide but instead find support, treatment, and other ways to cope—messages we want to focus on instead. The SAMHSA-funded National Action

Alliance for Suicide Prevention offers a Framework for Successful Messaging with specific tips on how to shift the focus from the problem of suicide to concrete steps for helping yourself and others plus stories of successful treatment and recovery.

- **Build relationships with reporters.** Share media guidelines, information about resources, and sample language with student reporters and local health and mental health reporters before a crisis occurs. If inappropriate coverage happens, contact the reporter or write an op-ed or letter to the editor.

SAMHSA's Recommendations For Reporting On Suicide

Important Points For Covering Suicide

- More than 50 research studies worldwide have found that certain types of news coverage can increase the likelihood of suicide in vulnerable individuals. The magnitude of the increase is related to the amount, duration, and prominence of coverage.

- Risk of additional suicides increases when the story explicitly describes the suicide method, uses dramatic/graphic headlines or images and repeated/extensive coverage sensationalizes or glamorizes a death.

- Covering suicide carefully, even briefly, can change public misperceptions and correct myths, which can encourage those who are vulnerable or at risk to seek help.

Suicide contagion or "copycat suicide" occurs when one or more suicides are reported in a way that contributes to another suicide.

Warning Signs Of Suicide:

- Talking about wanting to die
- Looking for a way to kill oneself
- Talking about feeling hopeless or having no purpose
- Talking about feeling trapped or in unbearable pain
- Talking about being a burden to others
- Increasing the use of alcohol or drugs
- Acting anxious, agitated, or recklessly
- Sleeping too little or too much

- Withdrawing or feeling isolated
- Showing rage or talking about seeking revenge
- Displaying extreme mood swings

The more of these signs a person shows, the greater the risk. Warning signs are associated with suicide, but may not be what causes a suicide.

What To Do

If someone you know exhibits warning signs of suicide:

- Do not leave the person alone.
- Remove any firearms, alcohol, drugs, or sharp objects that could be used in a suicide attempt.
- Call the U.S. National Suicide Prevention Lifeline at 800-273-TALK (800-273-8255).
- Take the person to an emergency room or seek help from a medical or mental health professional.

Suicide is a public health issue. Media and online coverage of suicide should be informed by using best practices. Some suicide deaths may be newsworthy. However, the way media cover suicide can influence behavior negatively by contributing to contagion or positively by encouraging help-seeking.

Table 44.1. Important Points For Media Coverage Of Suicide

Instead Of This	Do This
Big or sensationalistic headlines or prominent placement (e.g., Kurt Cobain Used Shotgun To Commit Suicide).	Inform the audience without sensationalizing the suicide and minimize prominence (e.g., Kurt Cobain Dead at 27).
Including photos/videos of the location or method of death, grieving family, friends, memorials, or funerals	Use school/work or family photo; include hotline logo or local crisis phone numbers.
Describing recent suicides as an epidemic, skyrocketing, or in other strong terms.	Carefully investigate the most recent CDC data and use non-sensational words like rise or higher.
Describing a suicide as inexplicable or without warning.	Most, but not all, people who die by suicide exhibit warning signs. Understand the warning signs and learn what to do in such cases.
John Doe left a suicide note saying….	A note from the deceased was found and is being reviewed by the medical examiner.

Table 44.1. Continued

Instead Of This	Do This
Investigating and reporting on suicide similar to reporting on crimes.	Report on suicide as a public health issue.
Quoting/interviewing police or first responders about the causes of suicide.	Seek advice from suicide prevention experts.
Referring to suicide as successful, unsuccessful, or a failed attempt.	Describe as died by suicide or completed or killed him/herself.

Avoid Misinformation And Offer Hope

- Suicide is complex. There are almost always multiple causes, including psychiatric illnesses, that may not have been recognized or treated. However, these illnesses are treatable.

- Refer to research findings that mental disorders and/or substance abuse have been found in 90 percent of people who have died by suicide.

- Avoid reporting that death by suicide was preceded by a single event, such as a recent job loss, divorce, or bad grades. Reporting like this leaves the public with an overly simplistic and misleading understanding of suicide.

- Consider quoting a suicide prevention expert on causes and treatments. Avoid putting expert opinions in a sensationalistic context.

- Use your story to inform readers about the causes of suicide, its warning signs, trends in rates, and recent treatment advances.

- Add statement(s) about the many treatment options available, stories of those who overcame a suicidal crisis and resources for help.

- Include up-to-date local/national resources where readers/viewers can find treatment, information, and advice that promotes help-seeking.

Suggestions For Online Media, Message Boards, Bloggers, And Citizen Journalists

- Bloggers, citizen journalists, and public commentators can help reduce risk of contagion with posts or links to treatment services, warning signs, and suicide hotlines.

- Include stories of hope and recovery, information on how to overcome suicidal thinking and increase coping skills.

- The potential for online reports, photos/videos, and stories to go viral makes it vital that online coverage of suicide follow site or industry safety recommendations.

- Social networking sites often become memorials to the deceased and should be monitored for hurtful comments and for statements that others are considering suicide. Message board guidelines, policies, and procedures could support removal of inappropriate and/or insensitive posts.

Chapter 45

Individual, Family, And Community Connectedness Help Prevent Suicidal Behavior

Over the past three decades, scientific research and conceptual thinking have converged to suggest that suicidal behavior results from a combination of genetic, developmental, environmental, physiological, psychological, social, and cultural factors operating through diverse, complex pathways. In 2001, multiple agencies and sectors collaborated on publication of the National Strategy for Suicide Prevention, designed as a comprehensive and integrated approach to addressing suicide as a public health problem. One of the National Strategy's primary aims is to promote opportunities and settings to enhance connectedness among persons, families, and communities.

What's It Mean?

Connectedness is a common thread that weaves together many of the influences of suicidal behavior and has direct relevance for suicide prevention. The Centers for Disease Control and Prevention (CDC) define connectedness as the degree to which a person or group is socially close, interrelated, or shares resources with other persons or groups. This definition encompasses the nature and quality of connections both within and between multiple levels of the social ecology, including

- connectedness between individuals;
- connectedness of individuals and their families to community organizations; and
- connectedness among community organizations and social institutions.

About This Chapter: This chapter includes text excerpted from "Promoting Individual, Family, And Community Connectedness To Prevent Suicidal Behavior," Centers for Disease Control and Prevention (CDC), July 10, 2013. Reviewed January 2017.

Connectedness Between Persons

At the level of individual connectedness, a very clear pathway is that in times of stress, the number and quality of social ties people have can directly influence their access to social support—regardless of whether that support is instrumental or emotional, actual or perceived. Received or perceived social support is hypothesized to decrease the threat-level appraisal of the experienced stress and increase a person's ability to cope with the stressful event or situation.

Close and supportive interpersonal relationships also appear to confer general psychological benefits independent of stress that increase physiologic functioning, such as cardiovascular, endocrine, and immune systems. This results in improved overall health and resistance to stress and disease. Close and supportive interpersonal relationships may also help to discourage maladaptive coping behaviors such as suicidal behaviors or substance use and by virtue of normative social influences encourage adaptive coping behaviors such as professional help-seeking.

Substantial evidence supports the view that connectedness between persons reduces risk of suicidal behavior. General measures of social integration (for example, number of friends, higher frequency of social contact, low levels of social isolation or loneliness) have been found to be protective against suicidal thoughts and behaviors, as documented in studies of adolescents and young and older adults.

> Connectedness between adolescents and their parents or families has been associated with decreased suicidal behaviors. Not surprisingly, disrupted social networks (for example, family discord, problems with friends, ending of a romantic relationship) have the expected opposite effect, significantly increasing the risk of suicidal behaviors and death.

Connectedness Of Individuals And Their Families To Community Organizations

The value of connectedness of individuals and families to community organizations has been less well studied. It nonetheless has the potential to decrease risk for suicidal behavior. Examples of relevant community organizations include schools, universities, places of employment, community centers, and churches or other religious or spiritual organizations. Connectedness of adolescents to their schools, for example, has been shown to protect against suicidal thoughts and behaviors.

Although the influence of such positive attachments on suicidal behavior needs to be better studied, many theoretical reasons support the idea that stronger connections to such groups may decrease suicidal behavior. For example, stronger connections can increase a person's sense of belonging or "mattering" to a group, a sense of personal value or worth, and access to a larger source of support. Thus persons have greater motivation and ability to cope adaptively in the face of adversity. In addition, group members often monitor each others' behavior, take responsibility for each others' well-being, and can offer or recommend assistance and support. By increasing a community's connectedness to—and responsibility for—individual members, that community is also more likely to mobilize collectively to meet its members' needs.

Connectedness Among Community Organizations And Social Institutions

In the broadest sense, connectedness among larger organizations, infrastructures, and agencies can help to prevent suicidal behavior. Although the value of stronger connections among such organizations and institutions needs improved research and understanding, schools, universities, and workplaces that use, for example, formal or informal screening strategies for suicide risk should have strong connections with agencies that can provide prevention or treatment service. Formal relationships between support services and referring organizations will help ensure not only referrals to accessible, high-quality services, but will also ensure that services are actually delivered. Moreover, better connection of helping-resource systems could promote client well-being, as in the case of the frequent disconnect between the primary healthcare system and the mental healthcare system.

Focus On Positive Connectedness

It should be noted that the focus here is the promotion of positive (that is, health promoting, protective) connectedness. Of course, not all social connections enhance health and well-being; some research suggests that too many dependents in a person's life can lead to role overload, which can increase psychological distress. Additionally—though not yet rigorously or broadly studied—known incidents of connectedness with negative social or normative influences have allegedly contributed to suicidal behavior (for example, suicide pacts, gang involvement). These are clearly not the types of connectedness that need strengthening. They provide nonetheless clear markers of risk in which positive connectedness interventions might be most needed or most beneficial. Thus, the goal is not simply to increase the number of social ties or connections among persons or groups, but to enhance availability of and access to supportive connections.

By supporting healthy interpersonal relationships (for example, family, peer, and marital relationships), and by encouraging communities to care about and care for their members, the population at large is likely to experience more positive health and well-being, resulting in lower risk of suicidal behavior. Further, these connections can remove social barriers to help-seeking by those in need, so persons contemplating or planning suicide would be less likely to engage in life threatening behaviors. And if the need for social connectedness is met in a person who has engaged in nonfatal suicidal behaviors, he or she is less likely to repeat the behavior. Following a suicide, positive social connections decrease the likelihood that survivors in the family and community will engage in suicidal behavior.

Key Areas For Promoting Connectedness And Preventing Suicidal Behavior

- Interrupting the development of fatal and nonfatal suicidal behavior
- Integrating approaches to preventing profound life stresses that may contribute to suicidal behavior and interpersonal violence
- Addressing vulnerable populations

Chapter 46

Goals Of The National Strategy For Suicide Prevention

What Is The 2012 National Strategy For Suicide Prevention?

The 2012 National Strategy for Suicide Prevention (the National Strategy) is the result of a joint effort by the Office of the U.S. Surgeon General and the National Action Alliance for Suicide Prevention (Action Alliance).

The National Strategy is a call to action that is intended to guide suicide prevention actions in the United States over the next decade. It outlines four strategic directions with 13 goals and 60 objectives that are meant to work together in a synergistic way to prevent suicide in the nation.

Why A National Strategy For Suicide Prevention?

Suicide is a serious public health problem that causes immeasurable pain, suffering, and loss to individuals, families, and communities nationwide. Many people may be surprised to learn that suicide was one of the top 10 causes of death in the United States in 2009. And death is only the tip of the iceberg. For every person who dies by suicide, more than 30 others attempt suicide. Every suicide attempt and death affects countless other individuals. Family members, friends, coworkers, and others in the community all suffer the long-lasting consequences of suicidal behaviors.

About This Chapter: This chapter includes text excerpted from "2012 National Strategy For Suicide Prevention: Goals And Objectives For Action," Substance Abuse and Mental Health Services Administration (SAMHSA), September 2, 2012. Reviewed January 2017.

Suicide places a heavy burden on the nation in terms of the emotional suffering that families and communities experience as well as the economic costs associated with medical care and lost productivity. And yet suicidal behaviors often continue to be met with silence and shame. These attitudes can be formidable barriers to providing care and support to individuals in crisis and to those who have lost a loved one to suicide.

Recognizing the importance of suicide prevention to the nation, in 2001 Surgeon General David Satcher released the first National Strategy for Suicide Prevention. This landmark document launched an organized effort to prevent suicide in the United States.

Activity in the field of suicide prevention has grown dramatically since the National Strategy was issued in 2001. Government agencies at all levels, schools, nonprofit organizations, and businesses have started programs to address suicide prevention. Important achievements include the enactment of the Garrett Lee Smith Memorial Act, the creation of the National Suicide Prevention Lifeline (800–273–TALK (800–273–8255)) and its partnership with the Veterans Crisis Line, and the establishment of the Suicide Prevention Resource Center (SPRC). Other areas of progress include the increased training of clinicians and community members in the detection of suicide risk and appropriate response, and enhanced communication and collaboration between the public and private sectors on suicide prevention.

Key Facts

- Suicide is the 10th leading cause of death, claiming more than twice as many lives each year as does homicide.

- On average, between 2001 and 2009, more than 33,000 Americans died each year as a result of suicide, which is more than 1 person every 15 minutes.

- More than 8 million adults report having serious thoughts of suicide in the past year, 2.5 million report making a suicide plan in the past year, and 1.1 million report a suicide attempt in the past year.

- Almost 16 percent of students in grades 9 to 12 report having seriously considered suicide, and 7.8 percent report having attempted suicide one or more times in the past 12 months.

Why Was The National Strategy Updated And Revised?

The National Strategy was revised to reflect major developments in suicide prevention, research, and practice during the past decade.

Examples include the following.

An increased understanding of the link between suicide and other health issues. Research confirms that health conditions such as mental illness and substance abuse, as well as traumatic or violent events can influence a person's risk of suicide attempts later in life. Research also suggests that connectedness to family members, teachers, coworkers, community organizations, and social institutions can help protect individuals from a wide range of health problems, including suicide risk.

New knowledge on groups at increased risk. Research continues to suggest important differences among various demographics in regards to suicidal thoughts and behaviors. This research emphasizes that communities and organizations must specifically address the needs of these communities when developing prevention strategies.

Evidence of the effectiveness of suicide prevention interventions. New evidence suggests that a number of interventions, such as behavior therapy and crisis lines, are particularly useful for helping individuals at risk for suicide. Social media and mobile apps provide new opportunities for intervention.

Increased recognition of the value of comprehensive and coordinated prevention efforts. Combining new methods of treating suicidal patients with a prompt patient follow-up after they have been discharged from the hospitals is an effective suicide prevention method.

How Is The National Strategy Organized?

The 2012 National Strategy for Suicide Prevention is closely aligned with the National Prevention Strategy, released in June 2011, which outlines the nation's plan for promoting better health and wellness among the population. This comprehensive plan seeks to increase the number of Americans who are healthy at every stage of life. Three of its seven priority areas—mental and emotional well-being, preventing drug abuse and excessive alcohol use, and injury- and violence-free living—are directly related to suicide prevention. Like the National Prevention Strategy, the 2012 National Strategy for Suicide Prevention recognizes that prevention should be woven into all aspects of our lives. Everyone—businesses, educators, healthcare institutions, government, communities, and every single American—has a role in preventing suicide and creating a healthier nation.

The National Strategy's goals and objectives fall within four strategic directions, which, when working together, may most effectively prevent suicides:

1. Create supportive environments that promote healthy and empowered individuals, families, and communities (4 goals, 16 objectives);

2. Enhance clinical and community preventive services (3 goals, 12 objectives);

3. Promote the availability of timely treatment and support services (3 goals, 20 objectives); and

4. Improve suicide prevention surveillance collection, research, and evaluation (3 goals, 12 objectives).

This organization represents a slight change from the AIM (Awareness, Intervention, Methodology) framework adopted in the 2001 National Strategy. The Awareness area has been included under Healthy and Empowered Individuals, Families, and Communities. The goals and objectives formerly included in the Intervention area have been spread across the first three strategic directions. Methodology has been expanded to include not only surveillance and research but also program evaluation. The 2001 goals and objectives have been updated, revised, and in some cases, replaced to reflect advances in knowledge and areas where the proposed actions have been completed.

Although some groups have higher rates of suicidal behaviors than others, the goals and objectives do not focus on specific populations or settings. Rather, they are meant to be adapted to meet the distinctive needs of each group, including new groups that may be identified in the future as being at an increased risk for suicidal behaviors.

What Are Some Of The Major Themes In The National Strategy?

Everyone has a role in preventing suicides. The goals and objectives in the National Strategy work together to promote wellness, increase protection, reduce risk, and promote effective treatment and recovery.

From encouraging dialogue about suicidal behavior to promoting policies that support suicide prevention, the National Strategy states that suicide prevention efforts should:

- Foster positive public dialogue, counter shame, prejudice, and silence; and build public support for suicide prevention;

- Address the needs of vulnerable groups, be tailored to the cultural and situational contexts in which they are offered, and seek to eliminate disparities;

- Be coordinated and integrated with existing efforts addressing health and behavioral health and ensure continuity of care;

- Promote changes in systems, policies, and environments that will support and facilitate the prevention of suicide and related problems;

- Bring together public health and behavioral health;

- Promote efforts to reduce access to lethal means among individuals with identified suicide risks; and

- Apply the most up-to-date knowledge base for suicide prevention.

Part Six
If You Need More Information

Chapter 47
Suicide And Crisis Hotlines

National (U.S.) Suicide Hotlines

Christian Suicide Hotline (CSP)
888-667-5947

Lesbian, Gay, Bisexual, Transgender and Questioning (LGBTQ) Suicide Hotline (the Trevor Lifeline)
866-488-7386
Available 24 hours a day, seven days a week

National Suicide Hopeline
800-SUICIDE (800-784-2433)

National Suicide Prevention Lifeline
800-273-TALK (800-273-8255)

Teen Suicide Hotline (Thursday's Child National Youth Advocacy Hotline)
800-USA-KIDS (800-872-5437)
Available 24 hours a day, seven days a week

Canadian Suicide Hotline

Distress/Suicide Help Line
800-232-7288 (Canada only)

Resources in this chapter were compiled from several sources deemed reliable; all contact information was verified and updated in January 2017.

Other Toll-Free Numbers For Suicide Prevention Information

American Foundation for Suicide Prevention (AFSP)
888-333-AFSP (888-333-2377)

Asian American Suicide Prevention and Education (AASPE)
877-990-8585
Available 24 hours a day, seven days a week

Jason Foundation, Inc. (JFI)
888-881-2323

Suicide Prevention Resource Center (SPRC)
877-GET-SPRC (877-438-7772)

Trevor Lifeline
866-488-7386

Other Crisis Hotlines

Al-Anon/Alateen Information Line
800-344-2666

National Youth Crisis Hotline
800-442-HOPE (800-442-4673)

Alcohol and Drug Help Line

WellPlace
800-821-HELP (800-821-4357)

Alcohol Hotline

Adcare Hospital
800-ALCOHOL (800-252-6465)

American Council on Alcoholism (ACA)
800-527-5344

ARK Crisis Line
800-873-TEEN (800-873-8336)

Boys Town National Hotline
800-448-3000

Center for Substance Abuse Treatment
800-662-HELP (800-662-4357) (English)
877-767-8432 (Spanish)
800-487-4889 (TDD)

Mood Disorders Support Group
212-673-3000
24 Hour Hotline

Nine Line

Covenant House Hotline
800-999-9999
7 days a week 1 p.m.–5 p.m.

Eating Disorder Awareness and Prevention

National Eating Disorders Association (NEDA)
800-931-2237
Monday-Thursday from 9 a.m. to 9 p.m. Eastern Time and Friday 9 a.m. to 5 p.m.

Narconon International Help Line
800-893-7060

NAMI Information Helpline

National Alliance on Mental Illness (NAMI)
800-950-NAMI (800-950-6264)

National Center For Missing And Exploited Children (NCMEC)
800-THE-LOST (800-843-5678)
24-hour call center

National Center For Victims Of Crime (NCVC)
800-FYI-CALL (800-394-2255)
8:30 a.m.–8:30 p.m. ET

National Child Abuse Hotline
Childhelp USA
800-4-A-CHILD (800-422-4453)

National Clearinghouse for Alcohol and Drug Information (NCADI)
800-729-6686
877-767-8432 (Spanish)
800-487-4889 (TDD)

National Domestic Violence Hotline
800-799-SAFE (800-799-7233)
800-787-3224 (TTY)

National Organization for Victim Assistance (NOVA)
800-TRY-NOVA (800-879-6682)
Monday–Friday 9:00 a.m.–5:00 p.m. ET

National Runaway Safeline (NRS)
800-RUNAWAY (800-786-2929)

National Sexual Assault Hotline
Rape, Abuse, and Incest National Network (RAINN)
800-656-HOPE (800-656-4673)

Operation Lookout National Center For Missing Youth
800-LOOKOUT (800-566-5688)

Stop It Now!
888-PREVENT (888-773-8368)

United Way Information Referral Service
800-233-HELP (800-233-4357)

Chapter 48

Agencies That Provide Information On Suicide And Mental Health

Government Agencies That Provide Information About Suicide

Center for Mental Health Services (CMHS)

Substance Abuse and Mental Health Services Administration (SAMHSA)
5600 Fishers Ln.
Rockville, MD 20857
Phone: 240-276-1310
Fax: 240-221-4295
Website: www.samhsa.gov/about-us/who-we-are/offices-centers/cmhs

Eunice Kennedy Shriver *National Institute of Child Health and Human Development (NICHD)*

P.O. Box 3006
Rockville, MD 20847
Toll-Free: 800-370-2943
TTY: 888-320-6942
Fax: 866-760-5947
Website: www.nichd.nih.gov
E-mail: NICHDInformationResourceCenter@mail.nih.gov

Resources in this chapter were compiled from several sources deemed reliable; all contact information was verified and updated in January 2017.

National Center for Post Traumatic Stress Disorder

(116D) VA Medical Center, 215 N. Main St.
White River Junction, VT 05009
Toll-Free: 844-MyVA311 (844-698-2311)
Phone: 802-296-5132
Fax: 802-296-5135
Website: www.ptsd.va.gov
E-mail: ncptsd@va.org

National Institute of Mental Health (NIMH)

6001 Executive Blvd.
Rm. 6200, MSC 9663
Bethesda, MD 20892-9663
Toll-Free: 866-615-NIMH (866-615-6464)
Phone: 301-443-4513
TTY: 301-443-8431
Toll-Free TTY: 866-415-8051
Fax: 301-443-4279
Website: www.nimh.nih.gov
E-mail: nimhinfo@nih.gov

National Institute on Alcohol Abuse and Alcoholism (NIAAA)

5635 Fishers Ln.
MSC 9304
Bethesda, MD 20892-9304
Phone: 301-443-3860
Website: www.niaaa.nih.gov
E-mail: niaaweb-r@exchange.nih.gov

National Institute on Drug Abuse (NIDA)

6001 Executive Blvd.
Rm. 5213, MSC 9561
Bethesda, MD 20892-9561
Phone: 301-443-1124
Website: www.drugabuse.gov

Office of Safe and Healthy Students (OSHS)

U.S. Department of Education (ED)
400 Maryland Ave. S.W.
Rm. 3E-245
Washington, DC 20202-6450
Phone: 202-453-6777
Fax: 202-453-6742
Website: www2.ed.gov/about/offices/list/oese/oshs/index.html
E-mail: OESE@ed.gov

Substance Abuse and Mental Health Services Administration (SAMHSA)

5600 Fishers Ln.
Rockville, MD 20857
Toll-Free: 877-SAMHSA-7 (877-726-4727)
Phone: 240-276-1310
Toll-Free TDD: 800-487-4889
Fax: 301-480-8491
Website: www.samhsa.gov

Private Agencies That Provide Information About Suicide

Al-Anon/Alateen Hot Line

1600 Corporate Landing Pkwy.
Virginia Beach, VA 23454-5617
Toll-Free: 800-344-2666
Phone: 757-563-1600
Fax: 757-563-1656
Website: www.al-anon.alateen.org
E-mail: wso@al-anon.org

American Academy of Child and Adolescent Psychiatry

3615 Wisconsin Ave. N.W.
Washington, DC 20016-3007
Phone: 202-966-7300
Fax: 202-464-0131
Website: www.aacap.org
E-mail: communications@aacap.org

American Association of Suicidology
5221 Wisconsin Ave. N.W.
Washington, DC 20015
Phone: 202-237-2280
Fax: 202-237-2282
Website: www.suicidology.org
E-mail: info@suicidology.org

American Foundation for Suicide Prevention
120 Wall St.
29th Fl.
New York, NY 10005
Toll-Free: 888-333-AFSP (888-333-2377)
Phone: 212-363-3500
Fax: 212-363-6237
Website: www.afsp.org
E-mail: info@afsp.org

American Group Psychotherapy Association
25 E. 21st St.
6th Fl.
New York, NY 10010
Phone: 212-477-2677
Fax: 212-979-6627
Website: www.agpa.org
E-mail: info@agpa.org

American Psychiatric Association
1000 Wilson Blvd.
Ste. 1825
Arlington, VA 22209-3901
Toll-Free: 888-35-PSYCH (888-357-7924)
Phone: 703-907-7300
Website: www.psychiatry.org
E-mail: apa@psych.org

American Psychiatric Nurses Association
Fairway Park Dr., Ste. 625
Falls Church, VA 22042
Toll-Free: 855-863-APNA (855-863-2762)
Phone: 571-533-1919
Fax: 855-883-APNA (855-883-2762)
Website: www.apna.org

American Psychological Association
750 First St. N.E.
Washington, DC 20002-4242
Toll-Free: 800-374-2721
Phone: 202-336-5500
TDD/TTY: 202-336-6123
Website: www.apa.org

American Psychotherapy Association
2750 E. Sunshine St.
Springfield, MO 65804
Toll-Free: 800-205-9165
Phone: 417-823-0173
Website: www.americanpsychotherapy.com

Anxiety and Depression Association of America
8701 Georgia Ave.
Ste. 412
Silver Spring, MD 20910
Phone: 240-485-1001
Fax: 240-485-1035
Website: www.adaa.org
E-mail: information@adaa.org

Association for Behavioral and Cognitive Therapies
305 7th Ave.
16th Fl.
New York, NY 10001
Phone: 212-647-1890
Fax: 212-647-1865
Website: www.abct.org

Association for Death Education and Counseling
1 Parkview Plaza
Ste. 800
Oakbrook Terrace, IL 60181
Phone: 847-686-2240
Fax: 847-686-2251
Website: www.adec.org
E-mail: adec@adec.org

The Brady Center to Prevent Gun Violence
840 First St. N.E.
Ste. 400
Washington, DC 20002
Toll-Free: 800-332-4483
Phone: 202-370-8101
Website: www.bradycampaign.org
E-mail: brady@bradymail.org

Centre for Addiction and Mental Health
33 Russell St.
Toronto, ON M5S 2S1
Canada
Toll-Free: 800-463-2338
Phone: 416-535-8501
Website: www.camh.ca

Depressed Anonymous
P.O. Box 17414
Louisville, KY 40217
Website: www.depressedanon.com
E-mail: depanon@netpenny.net

Depression and Bipolar Support Alliance (DBSA)
55 E. Jackson Blvd.
Ste. 490
Chicago, IL 60604
Toll-Free: 800-826-3632
Fax: 312-642-7243
Website: www.dbsalliance.org
E-mail: info@dbsalliance.org

Families for Depression Awareness
391 Totten Pond Rd., Ste. 101
Waltham, MA 02451
Phone: 781-890-0220
Fax: 781-890-2411
Website: www.familyaware.org
E-mail: info@familyaware.org

International OCD Foundation, Inc.
18 Tremont St.
Ste. 308
Boston, MA 02108
Phone: 617-973-5801
Fax: 617-973-5803
Website: www.iocdf.org
E-mail: info@iocdf.org

Jason Foundation
18 Volunteer Dr.
Hendersonville, TN 37075
Toll-Free: 888-881-2323
Phone: 615-264-2323
Fax: 615-264-0188
Website: www.jasonfoundation.com
E-mail: contact@jasonfoundation.com

Jed Foundation
6 E. 39th St.
Ste. 1204
New York, NY 10016
Phone: 212-647-7544
Fax: 212-647-7542
Website: www.jedfoundation.org

Mental Health America (MHA)
500 Montgomery St., Ste. 820
Alexandria, VA 22314
Toll-Free: 800-969-6642
Phone: 703-684-7742
Fax: 703-684-5968
Website: www.mentalhealthamerica.net

Mood Disorders Support Group

P.O. Box 30377
New York, NY 10011
Phone: 212-533-MDSG (212-533-6374)
Website: www.mdsg.org
E-mail: info@mdsg.org

National Alliance on Mental Illness (NAMI)

3803 N. Fairfax Dr., Ste. 100
Arlington, VA 22203
HelpLine: 800-950-6264
Phone: 703-524-7600
Website: www.nami.org
E-mail: info@nami.org

National Association for Children of Alcoholics (NACOA)

10920 Connecticut Ave., Ste. 100
Kensington, MD 2089
Toll-Free: 888-55-4COAS (888-554-2627)
Phone: 301-468-0985
Fax: 301-468-0987
Website: www.nacoa.org
E-mail: nacoa@nacoa.org

National Association of Anorexia Nervosa and Associated Disorders

750 E. Diehl Rd., Ste. 127
Naperville, IL 60563
Phone: 630-577-1330; 630-577-1333
Website: www.anad.org
E-mail: hello@anad.org

National Center for Victims of Crime

2000 M St. N.W., Ste. 480
Washington, DC 20036
Phone: 202-467-8700
Fax: 202-467-8701
Website: www.victimsofcrime.org
E-mail: webmaster@ncvc.org

National Center on Addiction and Substance Abuse at Columbia University

633 Third Ave.
19th Fl.
New York, NY 10017-6706
Phone: 212-841-5200
Website: www.centeronaddiction.org

National Coalition Against Domestic Violence (NCADV)

1 Bdwy.
Ste. B210
Denver, CO 80203
Phone: 303-839-1852
Fax: 303-831-9251
Website: www.ncadv.org
E-mail: mainoffice@ncadv.org

National Council on Alcoholism and Drug Dependence, Inc. (NCADD)

217 Bdwy.
Ste. 712
New York, NY 10007
Toll-Free: 800-NCA-CALL (800-622-2255)
Phone: 212-269-7797
Fax: 212-269-7510
Website: www.ncadd.org
E-mail: national@ncadd.org

National Eating Disorders Association (NEDA)

165 W. 46th St.
Ste. 402
New York, NY 10036
Toll-Free: 800-931-2237
Phone: 212-575-6200
Fax: 212-575-1650
Website: www.nationaleatingdisorders.org
E-mail: info@NationalEatingDisorders.org

National Empowerment Center (Recovery from Mental Illness)

599 Canal St.
Lawrence, MA 01840
Toll-Free: 800-power2u (800-769-3728)
Phone: 978-685-1494
Fax: 978-681-6426
Website: www.power2u.org
E-mail: info4@power2u.org

National Organization for People of Color Against Suicide (NOPCAS)

P.O. Box 75571
Washington, DC 20013
Phone: 973-204-8233
Website: www.nopcas.org

National Organization for Victim Assistance

510 King St.
Ste. 424
Alexandria, VA 22314
Toll-Free: 800-879-6682
Phone: 703-535-6682
Fax: 703-535-5500
Website: www.trynova.org

Other Mental Health Resources

S.A.F.E. ALTERNATIVES®

Toll-Free: 800-DONT-CUT (800-366-8288)
Fax: 888-296-7988
Website: www.selfinjury.com
E-mail: info@selfinjury.com

The Samaritans of New York

P.O. Box 1259
Madison Sq. Stn
New York, NY 10159
Phone: 212-673-3661
Website: www.samaritansnyc.org
E-mail: inquiries@samaritansnyc.org

Agencies That Provide Information On Suicide And Mental Health

SAVE—Suicide Awareness Voices of Education
8120 Penn Ave. S.
Ste. 470
Bloomington, MI 55431
Phone: 952-946-7998
Website: www.save.org

Suicide Prevention Resource Center
43 Foundry Ave.
Waltham, MA 02453
Toll-Free: 877-GET-SPRC (877-438-7772)
TTY: 617-964-5448
Website: www.sprc.org
E-mail: info@sprc.org

Treatment Advocacy Center
200 N. Glebe Rd.
Ste. 801
Arlington, VA 22203
Phone: 703-294-6001
Fax: 703-294-6010
Website: www.treatmentadvocacycenter.org
E-mail: info@treatmentadvocacycenter.org

Yellow Ribbon Suicide Prevention Program
7300 Lowell Blvd., Ste. 35
P.O. Box 644
Westminster, CO 80036
Toll-Free: 800-273-8255
Phone: 303-429-3530
Fax: 303-426-4496
Website: www.yellowribbon.org
E-mail: ask4help@yellowribbon.org

Chapter 49
Mobile Apps For Mental Health

Suicide Prevention

ASK & Prevent Suicide
This app helps to learn the warning signs and how to ask if someone is considering suicide.
Website: www.mhatexas.org/find-help

Calm in the Storm
This app helps to cope with the stresses of life. It can be customized to store experience and save the progress. Users can create their own safety plans.
Website: calminthestormapp.com

HELP Prevent Suicide
This app provides easy access to crisis intervention resources, including a list of warning signs, steps on how to talk with someone in crisis, and information on national and Oklahoma-specific resources.
Website: app.staplegun.us/help_prevent_suicide

Jason Foundation A Friend Asks
This app offers information, tools and resources to anyone who may be struggling with thoughts of suicide.
Website: jasonfoundation.com/get-involved/student/a-friend-asks-app

Lifebuoy
This is an interactive, self-help promoting app designed to assist suicide survivors as they normalize their lives after recent attempt.
Website: itunes.apple.com/us/app/lifebuoy-suicide-prevention/id686973252

Resources in this chapter were compiled from several sources deemed reliable; all contact information was verified and updated in January 2017.

MY3

This app helps to create support systems, build safety plans, and allows users to access National Suicide Prevention Lifeline 24/7.
Website: my3app.org

R U Suicidal?

This is a video-based, interactive self-help tool for anyone having thoughts about suicide.
Website: www.psychappsint.com

ReliefLink

This app is developed for suicide prevention and for improving mental health.
Website: itunes.apple.com/us/app/relieflink/id721474553

Suicide Lifeguard

This app is intended for anyone concerned that someone they know may be thinking of suicide. It provides information on warning signs of suicide, suicidal thoughts and/or intentions, and how to respond to them.
Website: www.mimhtraining.com/suicide-lifeguard

Suicide Safe by SAMHSA

This app is designed as a suicide prevention learning tool for primary care and behavioral health providers and is based on the nationally recognized Suicide Assessment Five-step Evaluation and Triage (SAFE-T) practice guidelines.
Website: store.samhsa.gov/apps/suicidesafe

Suicide Safety Plan

This app provides six evidence-based tools to aid against clinical depression and negative moods on a large scale.
Website: www.moodtools.org

TAPS

This app helps survivors connect with their peers and provide logistic updates during the event. This interactive tool will allow survivors to share stories and experiences, engage with Tragedy Assistance Program for Survivors (TAPS) through their social networks and post pictures of their favorite TAPS family events and activities—all in one place.
Website: www.taps.org/NMSSS/2016/MobileApp

You Are Important—Depression, Suicide and Bullying Prevention Videos App

This is a depression, suicide, and bullying prevention videos app.
Website: www.wonderiffic.com/you-are-important.htm

Depression

Depression CBT Self-Help Guide
This app is developed to offer self-help for depression
Website: www.excelatlife.com/apps.htm#depressionapp

iPrevail
This app is a safe and secure Peer support community helping others overcome anything that life sends their way.
Website: www.iprevail.com

Mood Sentry
This app designed to help porting of multiple computer based tools used to manage depression to a mobile platform.
Website: moodsentry.com

MoodMission
This is an evidence-based app designed to empower people to overcome low moods and anxiety by discovering new and better ways of coping.
Website: moodmission.com/app

WhatsMyM3
This app offers a 3 minute test for anxiety, bipolar disorder and PTSD
Website: www.whatsmym3.com

Anxiety

At Ease Anxiety and Worry Relief
This app is designed to relieve anxiety and worry by combining voice-guided breathing meditations, mental exercises and journaling.
Website: www.meditationoasis.com/at-ease-anxiety-worry-relief-app

Beat Panic
This app contains a series of flashcards designed in soothing colors and texts that assist in overcoming the panic attack in a gentle calm manner.
Website: itunes.apple.com/gb/app/beat-panic/id452656397

Breathe to Relax
This is portable stress management tool which provides detailed information on the effects of stress on the body and instructions and practice to help users learn the stress management skill called diaphragmatic breathing.
Website: t2health.dcoe.mil/apps/breathe2relax

eCBT Calm

This app provides a set of tools to help users to evaluate personal stress and anxiety, challenge distorted thoughts, and learn relaxation skills.
Website: ashfordu.readsh101.com/ecbt-calm

iCBT

This app is designed to help its users to manage stress and anxiety.
Website: itunes.apple.com/us/app/icbt/id355021834

MindShift

This app helps users to relax, develop more helpful ways of thinking, and identify active steps that will help to take charge of anxiety. It also includes strategies to deal with everyday anxiety.
Website: www.anxietybc.com/resources/mindshift-app

Pacifica

This app contains tools for stress and anxiety alongside a supportive community developed based on Cognitive Behavioral Therapy and meditation.
Website: www.thinkpacifica.com

Panic Attack Aid

This app is designed to bring instant calming relief from panic and anxiety attacks through breathing techniques, reassurance and distraction exercises.
Website: www.panic-attack-aid.com

Panic Relief

This app guides a person through panic attacks and helps to overcome fear.
Website: cognitivetherapyapp.com

Self-Help Anxiety Management

This app is designed to help its users understand and manage anxiety.
Website: sam-app.org.uk

Stress Tips

This app contains useful tips and advice on managing anxiety from volunteers, Anxiety UK staff, celebrity patrons and clinical advisors.
Website: www.anxietyuk.org.uk/our-services/mobile-app

WorryWatch

This is journal app to log and track anxiety.
Website: worrywatch.com

PTSD

CPT Coach

This is a treatment companion that helps its users and their therapist work through the CPT treatment manual.
Website: www.ptsd.va.gov/public/materials/apps/cpt_mobileapp_public.asp

PTSD Coach

This app helps to learn about and manage symptoms that often occur after trauma
Website: www.ptsd.va.gov/public/materials/apps/PTSDCoach.asp

Sleep

ChronoRecord

This app collects and analyzes data to increase the scientific understanding of mood disorders.
Website: chronorecord.org/html/home.html

iSleep Easy

This app contains a wide variety of guided meditations to help to fall asleep and sleep deeply.
Website: www.meditationoasis.com/isleep-easy-app

Pzizz Sleep

This is sleep and power nap system to fall asleep fast, stay asleep, and wake up feeling refreshed.
Website: pzizz.com

Relax Melodies

This apps is designed to help people who suffer from insomnia and other sleeping problems.
Website: www.ipnossoft.com/app/relax-melodies

Mood Charting

Mood Panda

This apps is designed to help people track their moods and to get anonymous support.
Website: www.moodpanda.com

MoodKit

This apps is designed to help users apply effective strategies of professional psychology to their everyday lives.
Website: www.thriveport.com/products/moodkit

MoodRhythm

This apps is designed to help patients with bipolar disorder monitor and analyze their daily rhythms and stay in balance.
Website: moodrhythm.com

My Life My Voice

This mood journal offers a simple solution for tracking thoughts, feelings, and moods.
Website: www.yourlifeyourvoice.org/Pages/mobile-app.aspx

Previdence

This is an evaluation tool that allows individuals to assess themselves or others for depression, anxiety, drug and alcohol and suicidal issues.
Website: itunes.apple.com/us/app/previdence/id506167832

Chapter 50
Online Resources For Suicide Survivors

American Association of Suicidiology

The American Association of Suicidiology offers education, training, and suicide prevention information. Click on "Suicide Loss Survivors" for a list of resources for people who have lost someone to suicide.
Website: www.suicidology.org

American Foundation for Suicide Prevention

AFSP, a non-profit organization, is involved in suicide-related research and suicide prevention. It also offers information for people whose lives have been touched by suicide. Other resources for suicide survivors include a bibliography of survivor guides, personal stories, and other books written for specific audiences.
Website: afsp.org

Compassionate Friends

Compassionate Friends offers help and support to grieving parents, siblings, and others following the death of a child from any cause, including suicide. The organization has chapters in all states.
Website: www.compassionatefriends.org

The Dougy Center

The Dougy Center provides structured peer support groups for children, teens, and young adults who have lost a parent, sibling, or friend as a result of suicide, homicide, accident, or illness.
Website: www.dougy.org

Resources in this chapter were compiled from several sources deemed reliable; all contact information was verified and updated in January 2017.

Friends and Families of Suicides

FFOS (Friends and Families of Suicides, which shares a website with Parents of Suicides) offers online support groups, memorial websites, and resources for people who have lost friends and family members by suicide.
Website: www.pos-ffos.com

International Association for Suicide Prevention

The International Association for Suicide Prevention works to help prevent suicides in different cultures around the world.
Website: www.iasp.info

Journey of Hearts

The Journey of Hearts website is designed to provide a place for people who are dealing with grief to receive support and information.
Website: journeyofhearts.org

The Link Counseling Center

The Link, a nonprofit counseling center, that offers confidential counseling, psychotherapy, and support groups to all ages.
Website: www.thelink.org

Suicide Prevention Action Network USA

SPAN USA is a division of the American Foundation for Suicide Prevention. It works to influence public policy.
Website: afsp.org

Survivors of Suicide

The SOS website was designed to help people deal with suicide bereavement.
Website: www.survivorsofsuicide.com

Index

Index

Page numbers that appear in *Italics* refer to tables or illustrations. Page numbers that have a small 'n' after the page number refer to citation information shown as Notes. Page numbers that appear in **Bold** refer to information contained in boxes within the chapters.

body dysmorphic disorder (BDD), self-esteem 259
body image
    anorexia nervosa 130
    self-esteem, overview 257–61
borderline personality disorder, overview 101–9
"Borderline Personality Disorder" (NIMH) 101n
Boys Town National Hotline, hotline 291
BPD see borderline personality disorder
brain
    BPD risk factors 103
    depression 65
    drug use 193
    mood stabilizers 184
    prescription drug abuse 117
    schizophrenia 95
brain function
    bipolar disorder 76
    opioids 118
brain stimulation therapy
    depression 64
    mental health disorders 173
    see also electroconvulsive therapy; repetitive transcranial magnetic stimulation; vagus nerve stimulation
Breathe to Relax, mobile app 307
Brady Center to Prevent Gun Violence
    contact 298
    publication
        suicide and guns truth 37n
bulimia nervosa, described 130
bully-victim, suicide 136
bullying
    anxiety disorders **83**
    LGBT youth 56
    sexual orientation 32
    suicide, overview 135–40
    suicide contagion prevention 272
    teen dating violence 121
    see also cyberbullying
bupropion
    antidepressants 174
    schizophrenia 93
buspirone
    anxiety disorders 177
    side effects 179

C

caffeine, stress management 85

Calm in the Storm, mobile app 305
CAMS see collaborative assessment and management of suicidality
catatonia, movement disorders 91
CBT see cognitive behavioral therapy
CDC see Centers for Disease Control and Prevention
Centre for Addiction and Mental Health, contact 298
Center for Mental Health Services (CMHS), contact 293
Center for Substance Abuse Treatment, hotline 291
Centers for Disease Control and Prevention (CDC)
    publications
        bullying and suicide in schools 135n
        children's mental health 237n
        dating violence 121n
        early start for schools 249n
        LGBT youth health study 51n
        mental health basics 45n
        preventing suicidal behavior 277n
        risk and protective factors 151n
        sleep habits 249n
        suicide prevention 15n
child abuse, described 123
"Child Abuse Leaves Epigenetic Marks" (NHGRI) 121n
childhood mental disorder, described 237
children
    bipolar disorders 75
    brain function 250
    bullying 135
    child abuse 122
    firearms 40
    mental health 46
    mental health disorder treatment 173
    PTSD **231**
    sexual abuse 31
    suicide statistics 5
    suicide survivors **214**
    trauma 225
"Children's Mental Health—New Report" (CDC) 237n
chlorpromazine, antipsychotic medications 181
Christian Suicide Hotline (CSP), hotline 289
ChronoRecord, mobile app 309
citalopram, antidepressants 174
clinical depression
    bulimia nervosa 132
    suicide loss 209
clonazepam, anti-anxiety medications 177

firearms, *continued*
   signs of suicide **104**, **274**
   suicidal link 39
   suicidal thoughts 246
   suicide statistics **5**, 10
"First National Study Of Lesbian, Gay, And Bisexual High School Students' Health" (CDC) 51n
flashbacks, trauma response 226
flooding, drugs of abuse 194
fluoxetine 174
fluphenazine 181
friends
   bipolar disorder 75
   body dysmorphic disorder 259
   body image 257
   dating violence 121
   depression 67, 70, 263
   drug addiction 195
   grieving process 222, **226**
   mental illness recovery 50
   peer counseling 230
   psychotherapy 78
   recovery process 157
   schizophrenia support 99
   signs of mental illness **238**
   signs of suicide 267
   social anxiety disorder 83
   social support 215
   stress factors 241
   suicidal risk **278**
   suicidal thoughts 144
   suicide contagion **234**
   suicide impact **213**, 245
   suicide prevention 281
   suicide prevention goals 274
   treatment support 48
Friends and Families of Suicides, website address 312

G

gender factor
   drug addiction 195
   eating disorders 132
   firearms 41
   suicidal behavior 29
   suicide statistics 26, 246
generalized anxiety disorder
   described 81
   medications 86, 177

generic medication, depression 72
genes
   bipolar disorder 76
   child abuse 123
   drug addiction 195
   eating disorders 132
   mental health problems 47
   schizophrenia 94
   traumatic childhood experiences 246
"Going To Therapy" (OWH) 165n
grief
   coping strategies, overview 219–23
   death 146
   friends 230
   overview 211–7
   peer counseling 230
   sudden loss 206
   support **226**
   trauma 230
   vicarious trauma **214**
   see also normal grief; complicated grief
"Grief, Bereavement, And Coping With Loss (PDQ®)—Patient Version" (NCI) 211n
group therapy
   borderline personality disorder 105
   defined 167
   social anxiety disorder 84
   see also Systems Training for Emotional Predictability and Problem Solving
guns *see* firearms

H

hallucinations
   antipsychotic medications 97, 181
   common grief 212
   described 90
   mood stabilizer side effects 185
   schizophrenia 92
   serotonin syndrome 176
   see also depression
haloperidol 181
"Having Body Image Issues" (OWH) 257n
heavy episodic drinking (HED), suicide research 33
HED *see* heavy episodic drinking
HELP Prevent Suicide, mobile app 305
"Helping Children And Adolescents Cope With Violence And Disasters: What Parents Can Do" (NIMH) 225n

R

S